A DENTAL PRACTITIONER HANDBOOK
SERIES EDITED BY DONALD D. DERRICK, DDS, LDS RCS

# AN INTRODUCTION TO FIXED APPLIANCES

K. G. ISAACSON

FDS, DOrth, RCS

*Consultant Orthodontist
to the Oxford Regional Health Authority
and to the Wessex Regional Health Authority*

and

J. K. WILLIAMS

BDS, FDS, DOrth, RCS

*Consultant Orthodontist
to the Leeds Regional Health Authority
and to the Dental Hospital at Leeds*

*Second edition*
With a Foreword by
Professor W. J. B. HOUSTON

BRISTOL: JOHN WRIGHT & SONS LTD
1978

CIP Data

Isaacson, Keith Geoffrey
    An introduction to fixed appliances. – 2nd ed. –
    ('Dental practitioner' handbooks; no. 17).
    1. Orthodontic appliances
    I. Title   II. Williams, John Kay   III. Series
    617.6'43'0028                    RK 527

    ISBN 0–7236–0480–0

*First edition,* 1973
*Second edition,* 1978

Text set in 11pt Photon Times, printed by photolithography, and bound in Great Britain at The Pitman Press, Bath

# PREFACE

A consideration of fixed-appliance techniques available at the present time will reveal a small number of clearly defined systems, which require the application of particular diagnostic criteria and which define treatment objectives. Some orthodontists are wholly committed to one or another of these techniques, and this polarization of opinion would suggest that no single technique is applicable to all cases. No doubt further refinements of mechanism will be developed, but they will arise out of experience gained by using existing methods. An understanding of the way in which simple fixed-appliance systems work is therefore important.

The authors of this book have two objectives. The first is to describe methods of moving teeth with fixed appliances which have proved to be successful in their hands. The second is to attempt to explain, compare, and contrast some basic principles of fixed-appliance work. The book is not a substitute for a formal course of instruction such as that leading to the examination for the Diploma in Orthodontics. It is intended to be complementary to such a course and also to be of interest to practitioners experienced with removable appliances. Diagnosis for the orthodontic patient is intentionally omitted from this book, and some aspects of fixed-appliance work which have been described in standard orthodontic textbooks are not included, but appropriate references are provided.

If this book can stimulate an interest in the basic principles which determine the movement of teeth with fixed appliances then it will have satisfied our intentions.

*Reading and Leeds, 1978*

K.G.I.
J.K.W.

# CONTENTS

# FOREWORD

By W. J. B. Houston

FDS RCS (EDIN), PHD, DORTH.
*Professor of Orthodontics, Royal Dental Hospital of
London School of Dental Surgery*

The demand for orthodontic treatment is increasing and patients are expecting higher standards of orthodontic care. While some malocclusions can be treated adequately by planned extractions and the use of removable appliances, in many cases fixed appliance treatment is essential if an optimal result is to be obtained. It is important that the general practitioner with a particular interest in orthodontics, the dentist who contemplates postgraduate training in order to specialize, and the postgraduate who has just commenced his training, should all have access to information about the basic principles that are common to every fixed appliance technique. It is these that this handbook expounds so clearly and thus should help to satisfy a need that has not otherwise been met. The subject is covered in sufficient scope and detail to satisfy the general practitioner and at the same time to provide an excellent foundation for the further studies of those who wish to specialize in orthodontics.

# CHAPTER 1

# INTRODUCTION

There are many factors which determine the nature of achieved tooth movement. One of these factors is the type of appliance used.

Removable appliances produce tooth movement essentially by tipping the teeth. In order to produce rotational, bodily, and apical movement efficiently, fixed appliances are required. A basic difference between the possibilities of tooth movement offered by removable and fixed appliances is thus immediately obvious.

A large number of fixed-appliance techniques are available, and the type of mechanism used will in part determine the nature of the tooth movement achieved.

This book describes ways in which tooth movement can be achieved using relatively simple appliances. Most of the techniques depend upon the use of round-wire arches. The principles involved are an extension of those used when treating a case with removable appliances. In situations where a removable appliance will produce the required tooth movement more efficiently than a fixed appliance, its use is recommended and described.

The book is therefore concerned mainly with mechanisms designed to produce given tooth movements. The exercise of diagnosis and treatment planning without the ability to move the teeth into the prescribed positions is useless. Likewise, the wholly mechanistic approach, and the reduction of occlusal relationships to 'norms', with scant attention to diagnosis, is inappropriate.

The interrelation of diagnosis and appliance method is important to recognize. It is often possible to formulate more than one treatment plan in a given case. The best plan is not necessarily that which will give an 'ideal' occlusal result. Economic and social factors and the potentialities of the appliance systems available, as well as the operator's ability must be taken into consideration.

CHAPTER 2

# THE SCOPE OF FIXED APPLIANCES

A comparison between the various orthodontic tooth movements that are possible and the method of applying a force in order to achieve these movements, will illustrate the potential of fixed appliances and the limitations of removable appliances. The movements that are to be considered are tipping, uprighting and torqueing, bodily movement and rotation.

*Tipping*

Tipping is the simplest tooth movement to carry out and is achieved by the application of a force to the crown of a tooth. The tooth moves under the influence of the force in the direction of least resistance. A fulcrum is established (usually within the root of the tooth) such that the crown moves in the direction of the applied force and the apex in the opposite direction. As the tooth moves, the location of the fulcrum influences the degree of angular change in the long axis of the tooth. The closer the fulcrum lies to the apex, the less the angular change for a given crown movement. The quality of movement is illustrated in *Fig.* 2.1. Removable appliances produce tooth movement principally

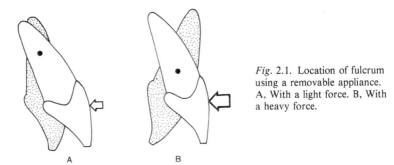

*Fig.* 2.1. Location of fulcrum using a removable appliance. A, With a light force. B, With a heavy force.

A                    B

by tipping, forces being applied by means of relatively simple springs acting directly upon the crowns of the teeth being moved.

The location of the fulcrum is influenced by:

1. The point of application of the force. If the point of application moves gingivally, the fulcrum moves apically. In practice, it is virtually impossible to maintain a constant point of application when using removable appliances.

2

2. The magnitude of the force applied. The ideal ('physiological') tipping force of 25–40 g for a single root is said to be associated with a fulcrum which lies near the junction between the apical one-third, and gingival two-thirds of the root. The use of higher forces produces movement of the fulcrum in a coronal direction, and therefore proportionally greater movement of the apex for a given crown movement.

Many malocclusions cannot be satisfactorily treated by means of tipping teeth in the manner described above. Furthermore, the location of the fulcrum when tipping teeth using removable appliances is not accurately predictable and is liable to change during tooth movement.

Fixed appliances are also capable of producing tipping movements, but their advantage over removable appliances is that by applying a force-couple to the crown of the tooth, controlled apical movement is possible.

### Uprighting and Torqueing

Both uprighting and torqueing involve controlled movement of the apices of teeth. In this book intentional mesial or distal movement of apices is referred to as uprighting, and labial or palatal movement of incisor apices is referred to as torqueing. Both uprighting and torqueing require the application of a force-couple to the crown in such a way that the fulcrum lies within the crown (*Fig.* 2.2).

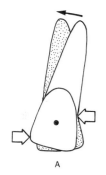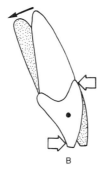

*Fig.* 2.2. A, Uprighting. B, Torqueing.

A        B

### Bodily Movement

Bodily movement of teeth implies an equal movement of crown and apex in the same direction. It is not possible to move a tooth bodily by means of a force applied to the crown unless the tooth is prevented from tipping. A fixed appliance can be designed in such a way that a force-couple is applied to the crown so that the apex moves in the same direction as the crown (*Fig.* 2.3A).

3

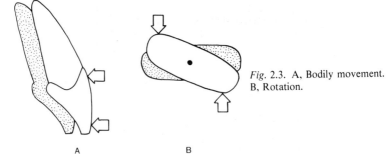

*Fig.* 2.3. A, Bodily movement. B, Rotation.

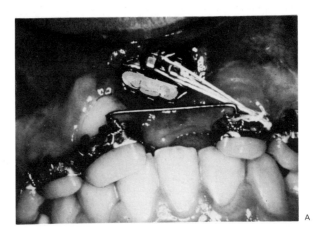

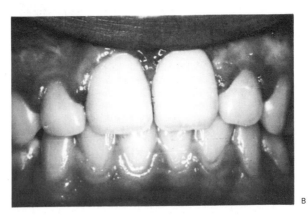

*Fig.* 2.4. A, A fixed appliance to align a labially displaced central incisor. B, Completion of treatment.

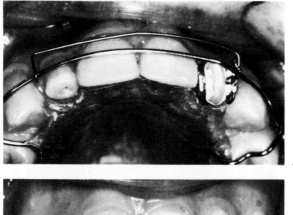

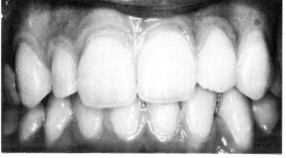

*Fig.* 2.5. Derotation of a lateral incisor with a band and whip spring to a removable appliance. A, Commencement of treatment. B, Completion of treatment.

## Rotation

Rotation of teeth around their long axis requires the application of a force-couple to the crown. There is considerable mechanical difficulty in applying an efficient force-couple with a removable appliance, but if the tooth requiring to be rotated is banded, precise rotational control can be obtained (*Fig.* 2.3B).

### *Specific Indications for the Use of Fixed Appliances*

### *Grossly Misplaced Teeth*

When the crown or apex of a tooth is markedly displaced from its correct position, particularly when movement in an occlusal direction is required, fixed appliances are necessary. If the displaced tooth is banded, a site is thereby provided for the application of forces (*Fig.* 2.4).

5

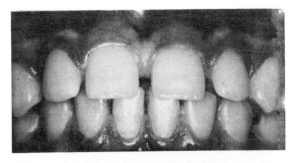

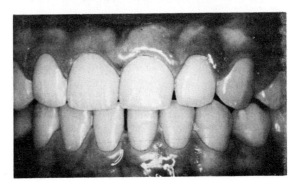

*Fig.* 2.6. Incisor spacing closed by a fixed appliance.

### Lower Arch Treatment

Lower removable appliances are not in general found to be satisfactory for the correction of other than very minor tooth displacement. They are bulky, tend to have poor retention and because of the restricted amount of space available cannot accommodate efficient springs. Lower fixed appliances, however, are mechanically satisfactory and can be used in conjunction with upper arch treatment by means of elastic intermaxillary traction.

### Rotated Teeth

The precise control over tooth position which is possible when using fixed appliances enables rotation to be readily achieved. A further advantage of using fixed appliances in this connection is that the abnormality of apical position so frequently associated with rotated teeth can be corrected simultaneously (*Fig.* 2.5).

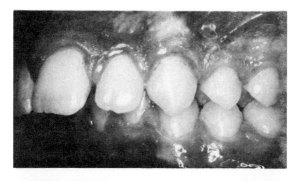

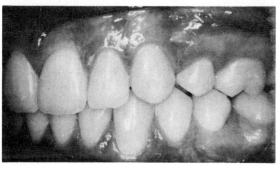

*Fig.* 2.7. An overjet reduced by a fixed appliance giving controlled apical movement.

## Space Closure

Space closure can be achieved using removable appliances, but only by means of tipping teeth into contact. Apart from the possible aesthetic and functional disadvantages, such movement is liable to relapse because of the failure to correct the apical positions of the teeth. When a fixed appliance is used, apical as well as coronal correction can be achieved. Controlled space closure is necessary for the treatment of spaced malocclusions, for example midline diastema (*Fig.* 2.6).

## Incisor Relationship

In certain Class II, division 1 malocclusions, an increased overjet is associated with a relatively severe skeletal 2 dental base relationship. If the overjet is reduced in such cases using removable appliances, because the upper incisors tip, they may well be excessively retroclined at the completion of treatment. This relationship can lead to an increased overbite, the lower incisors not occluding with the mid-

7

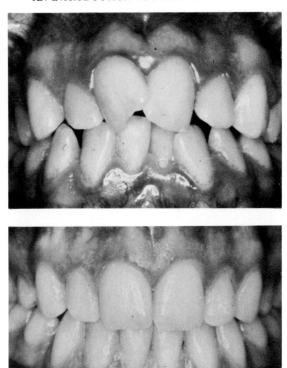

*Fig.* 2.8. Multiple rotations corrected by a fully banded fixed appliance.

dle third of palatal surface of the upper incisors, and a traumatic relationship may result. Fixed appliances, by virtue of the fact that they can control apical movement, can be used to reduce an overjet without excessive tipping, thereby producing a satisfactory interincisal relationship (*Fig.* 2.7). Severe Class II, division 2 incisor relationship and bimaxillary proclination of incisors can only be corrected by using fixed appliances, because of the necessity of altering the apical position of both the upper and lower incisors in order to achieve a stable change in the interincisal angle.

*Multiple Tooth Movement*

Fixed appliances allow for control over the position of several teeth or groups of teeth in either or both arches. Simultaneous tipping, rotation and apical movements are possible and both intermaxillary and extra-oral forces can be efficiently applied (*Fig.* 2.8).

# CHAPTER 3

# SUPERVISION OF THE PATIENT

The management of fixed appliances is demanding of the operator, and the wearing of a fixed appliance is no less demanding of the patient. For this reason it is important to ensure that it is the patient himself who wants the treatment to be undertaken. The orthodontist must approach the malocclusion as part of a living patient; otherwise there is a likelihood that the treatment will be a failure. The orthodontist must make an assessment of the following points before beginning treatment:

*Attitude of the Patient*

A significant cause of failure in orthodontic treatment is lack of motivation on the part of the patient. It is important not to embark upon a course of treatment which the patient feels is unnecessary. In the first instance, the orthodontist should discuss treatment aims with the prospective patient, without the parents being present. In this way, mutual respect can be established, in fact must be established, if the desired treatment result is to be identified and achieved.

*Oral Hygiene*

An excellent standard of oral hygiene must be maintained throughout treatment. It is of no use merely to instruct the patient of this when the appliance is cemented. The patient should demonstrate that he is able to maintain an adequate standard of oral hygiene before active treatment is begun. If a patient is unable to clean his teeth properly before treatment, he will find it even more difficult to do so with a complicated appliance in place. If oral hygiene is poor during the period of appliance wear, the possibility of decalcification and caries is greatly increased and periodontal problems made more severe. Instruction in plaque control and the correct use of a suitable toothbrush is of particular importance once the appliance is in place. The use of disclosing tablets is helpful in identifying areas of inadequate cleaning.

*Implications of Appliance Wear*

It is unfair to cement a fixed appliance without first explaining to the patient what the appliance is like, how it will feel, and how long it will have to be worn. It is not only unfair, it may also be expensive and time-consuming for the orthodontist because the patient may refuse to continue wearing the appliance for one reason or another.

Appearance is often a matter of great importance to the patient. A photograph of a patient wearing a fixed appliance is invaluable in demonstrating the appearance of a fixed appliance.

The question of pain may also arise. It should be explained to the patient that a certain amount of discomfort is involved, but that this is seldom a reason for a patient requesting removal of the appliance.

### Co-operation

The co-operation of the patient throughout treatment is, of course, essential. As well as attention to oral hygiene, the patient must understand the necessity for carrying out special instructions regarding the appliance. If the patient is unable or unwilling to do this, he is unsuitable for appliance treatment.

Good co-operation can often be obtained if the patient has an understanding of what is being achieved at each stage of treatment. An attempt should be made to make the patient consciously aware of the way in which the appliance functions.

### Attendance

Regular attendance throughout the treatment period is essential. Appointments will usually have to be made at intervals of approximately 4 weeks. Patients who are unwilling or unable to fulfil this requirement are not suitable for appliance treatment. If a fixed appliance is left unattended for a long period it may well produce unwanted tooth movement. It is important also that a patient should attend as soon as possible if the appliance becomes distorted or broken.

### Medical History

The patient's general medical condition must, of course, be taken into account before commencing orthodontic treatment.

## PREPARATION PRIOR TO THE FITTING OF A FIXED APPLIANCE

### Examination of the Teeth

Some time before band making a careful examination of the teeth should be made. Any carious cavities must be restored before band cementation. Discoloured teeth should be checked for vitality, and radiographs examined for any periapical pathology, shortening of the roots, or dilaceration.

Hypocalcified or decalcified areas on teeth, as well as stains, chipped incisal edges, and short roots, should be pointed out to the patient, and in the case of a young patient, to his parents. Any such abnormality should be recorded in the patient's notes.

It is emphasized that adequate radiographs must be available in order that the position and condition of both erupted and unerupted teeth can be verified.

## Preparation of the Mouth before Banding

It is a good plan to scale and polish the teeth thoroughly a few days before band making. Apart from the undesirability of calculus deposits from the periodontal standpoint, gross supragingival deposits make adequate band making impossible.

Fixed appliances, even when perfectly managed, are liable to cause deterioration in the condition of the periodontal tissues. An examination of the periodontal condition should therefore be made before treatment with fixed appliances, and advice or treatment for periodontal problems sought. In some cases periodontal conditions are directly associated with malocclusion and it may not be possible to resolve these problems before orthodontic treatment. Periodontal considerations must be borne in mind during treatment, when correct appliance design and proper oral hygiene are of great importance.

During orthodontic treatment with fixed appliances there is a danger of carious lesions developing under bands, due to faulty band adaptation, incorrect cementation, and loosening of bands. In addition, enamel decalcification may occur adjacent to bands because of inadequate oral hygiene. Whatever the cause there is a risk of caries, and for this reason topical application of fluroide gel before band cementation is used as a preventative measure. It has been suggested that when direct bonded attachments are used (p. 23), and areas of tooth surface therefore not protected by bands, that these surfaces are at added risk because the archwire further impedes adequate oral hygiene procedures. The daily use of fluoride-containing mouth rinses, and fluoride toothpaste may be particularly beneficial in these circumstances.

Following the removal of the appliance the teeth should again be scaled and polished, and a careful check kept on the periodontal condition.

## Records

Adequate records must be taken before treatment is commenced. These will often be available from the diagnosis and treatment planning stage. They include radiographs and reference models, which must be carefully stored. The reference models should be available at each appointment. Intra-oral, full-face, and profile photographs may be considered in order to complete the records.

## TREATMENT SUPERVISION

*Initial Archwire Fitting*

After a fixed appliance has been fitted, the patient must be instructed as to its care, and to watch carefully for breakages and distortion. It is advisable to have a printed series of instructions such as the following for the patient to take away and refer to at home:

### Care of Fixed Appliances

1. The appliance is fixed to your teeth and you must not attempt to remove or adjust it.

2. Initially it will cause some discomfort. This should not be severe, but if you are in doubt contact the orthodontist.

3. Sticky sweets, chewing gum, toffee, hard foods, tough meat, etc., can damage the appliance, so please do not eat them.

4. The appliance itself cannot harm the teeth, but damage will occur if it is not kept perfectly clean. The teeth and appliance must be cleaned gently but thoroughly after each meal and just before going to bed.

5. It is vital that any special instructions, such as the wearing of elastics or headgear, should be strictly followed.

6. In an emergency—if a band becomes loose or the appliance is damaged or painful—telephone . . . and an appointment will be arranged for you as soon as possible.

7. You must continue to see a dental surgeon every 4–6 months in order that any fillings which are required can be attended to.

The discomfort that a patient may experience following the fitting of a fixed appliance arises from:

*a.* Forces applied to the teeth by the appliance. These should, of course, never be excessive, and should be kept as low as possible for the first appointment.

*b.* The presence of bands and attachments which cause soreness of the mucous membrane of the lips, cheeks, and gingivae. This discomfort will decline as the wearing of the appliance continues. Soft red ribbon wax may be given to the patient to apply to the appliance where it is abrading the soft tissues.

*Subsequent Attendance*

At every visit it is advisable to follow a routine:

1. Ask the patient if there is anything wrong with the appliance, and check every band to see that it is not loose and that the cement has not become washed out between the band and the tooth. Even

with this care, some operators prefer to remove all the bands and re-cement them at 6–9-monthly intervals. This precaution is necessary in order to reduce the risk of decalcification under the bands.

2. Archwire. Even if the archwire is not removed from the mouth but just reactivated, it should be checked to see that it has not become obviously distorted.

3. Caries. Teeth carrying bands should be regularly checked for caries and treated accordingly. An arrangement must be made for the patient to have routine conservative treatment. In addition, the importance of a high standard of oral hygiene should be continually stressed, and an observation of the periodontal condition maintained.

4. When using fixed appliances, teeth which are being moved demonstrate an increased mobility and are often slightly tender. Any complaint of pain and any excessive tooth mobility must be investigated.

### Measurement and Observation

It is only by careful observation and measurement of tooth position that cases under orthodontic treatment can be properly supervised. The control of the amount of space available is particularly dependent upon careful measurement visit by visit, and measurements should be recorded in the patient's notes.

The distances between anchor teeth and the teeth being moved should be measured with dividers and ruler. Although a change in distance between two teeth is an indication of movement, this may not necessarily be a desirable movement. The teeth must be examined in occlusion, the overjet measured, and the molar and canine relationships compared with the patient's study models.

The position of the teeth in the buccal segment can then be related to the labial segments; however, during treatment the angulation of both the upper and lower labial segments can change. Although marked alterations in incisor angulation can be seen clinically, a lateral skull radiograph taken using a cephalostat is the only way in which these changes can be measured. For many cases a clinical estimation is adequate, but a lateral skull radiograph is necessary for a more precise assessment of the position of the teeth in both the buccal and labial segments.

### REFERENCES

Eastoe J. E., Picton D. C. A. and Alexander A. G. (1971) *The Prevention of Periodontal Disease*. London, Kimpton.
Silverstone L. M. (1976) *Dent. Update* **3,** 107.
Zachrisson B. U. (1976) *Am. J. Orthod.* **69,** 285.

# CHAPTER 4

# CASE PREPARATION

Careful attention to detail during band and bracket fitting is essential to enable a satisfactory treatment result to be obtained. Care must be taken in placing the band correctly, but it is the precise relationship of the brackets to the teeth that is of vital importance.

One of the drawbacks of fixed appliances is the possibility of decalcification, or even caries, of the teeth as the result of wearing bands. Decalcification may occur under bands where the cement has become washed away, and also in the gaps between the edges of the bands and the gingival margins of the teeth. Bands must as far as possible be self-retentive and close fitting. The height of the bands on the teeth is important; they should be in such a position that the brackets can be placed on the bands with the archwire channel about 3–4 mm from the occlusal surface of the tooth. Bands should not extend on to the occlusal surface of the tooth, or occlude with the teeth in the opposing arch.

## BAND FITTING

*Separation*

In many cases the fitting of bands is difficult because of the tightness of the interdental contact points. Where these contacts are very tight, it may be difficult or impossible to force the band far enough in a gingival direction and the band may become distorted in the attempt. Furthermore, tightness at the interproximal area may give the false impression of a tightly fitting band. Slight separation of the teeth between the contact points is obtained using separators.

MOLAR SEPARATION: Soft brass wire of 0·5 or 0·6 mm diameter is passed around the contact point. The two ends are then twisted tightly together, the excess cut off, and the twisted end tucked inwards (*Fig. 4.1*). Such separating wires should not be left in place for more than a week as they may work loose and become displaced. Separation can be maintained with preformed C-shaped separators.

Preformed separating springs or elastics are available for molar and premolar separation.

INCISOR SEPARATION: Separation is often needed, particularly for the lower incisors, and for this a preformed elastic strip, which is dumb-bell shaped in cross-section, is used. Short lengths are cut off the strip,

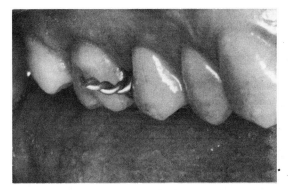

*Fig.* 4.1. Brass separating wire for molar separation. The twisted end is tucked in gingivally.

and the patient is instructed to place these between the contact points 2–3 hours before the appointment.

### Band-making

Bands may be made from stainless-steel tape which is contoured using band-forming pliers to fit the teeth in the mouth. Making individual bands in this manner is time consuming, and most operators are now using preformed bands. (For a description of band-making, *see* Beresford, 1966 and Graber, 1966.)

### Band Selection

Commercially produced preformed bands are now available, and in most instances give as good a fit as a band which has been pulled up by the operator. In addition, the fitting of preformed bands is more comfortable for the patient.

When choosing a band the study models may be used as a rough guide to the size of band required for a particular tooth, but band selection becomes easier with experience of a particular make of band. It is worthwhile noting (in the patient's notes) the size number of the band chosen for each tooth for future reference in case a band is mutilated beyond repair.

Bands are seated using band seating instruments which are applied to the occlusal edge of the bands. Certain bands have seating lugs that are attached to their palatal, or lingual aspects.

### Band Position

MOLAR AND PREMOLAR BANDS: The ideal position for a molar or premolar band is for the edge to rest just under the gingival margin without causing any blanching of the gingiva. In adults, because the

15

clinical crown is longer than it is in children, it is sometimes not possible to seat the band below the gingival margin of the tooth. Care must then be taken to see that the gap between the band and the gingival margin is not a small one, because this would be difficult to clean and give rise to decalcification. The band should not extend on to the occlusal surface of the tooth, or the band will soon be loosened by occlusal forces.

CANINE BANDS: The shape of a canine crown is such that, in order to achieve adequate retention, the band needs to be seated further gingivally than on the premolars or incisors. Canine bands therefore require a labial extension, or apron, for attachment of the bracket at the correct height from the cusp tip.

INCISOR BANDS: Incisor bands are fitted approximately in the middle of the crown, but the bands on upper lateral incisors require to be slightly nearer the incisal edge of the tooth. The incisal edge is not always a good guide to the position of the band, especially if the tooth is fractured. Incisor bands must be very carefully contoured to the tooth surface occlusally and gingivally because any decalcification will be obvious when the bands are removed.

BANDS ON PARTIALLY ERUPTED TEETH: Partially erupted teeth present a problem for band fitting, and it is useful to refer to the size of band used for the same tooth on the other side of the arch. When a tooth is only partially erupted and a band is difficult to seat fully, an attachment can be bonded directly to the tooth surface (*see* p. 23).

## BRACKETS AND ATTACHMENTS

### *Brackets*

The brackets most commonly used by the authors are edgewise and Begg brackets (*Fig.* 4.2).

Edgewise brackets are available in a wide range of size and design. They are broadly divisible into two types, the single edgewise bracket and the double, or Siamese, edgewise bracket. Siamese brackets are available in a variety of widths, so that suitable brackets are available for narrow lower incisors and for wide upper central incisors. Siamese brackets provide a considerable mesiodistal width for attachment to the archwire. Edgewise brackets are available with different sized archwire channels. The commonly used sizes are 0·45 mm and 0·55 mm.

Various patterns of Begg bracket are obtainable from manufacturers, but they are all basically similar. The Begg bracket carries a narrow slot into which the archwire is loosely fitted and held by a locking pin.

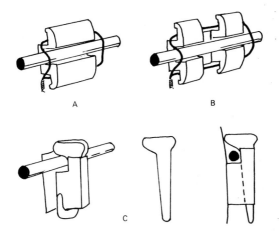

*Fig.* 4.2. A, Single edgewise bracket. B, Siamese edgewise bracket. C, Begg bracket and Begg pin.

*Bracket Position*

Bands may be purchased with the brackets and attachments prewelded in position. Alternatively, the brackets can be spotwelded in position by the operator. Care should be taken to ensure a firm attachment between brackets and bands, because if a bracket becomes loose the band must be removed and recemented. As a rule the brackets should be placed in the centre of the labial surface of the teeth, equidistant from the mesial and distal edges of the tooth. With rotated teeth it is often impossible to place the bracket in the middle of the buccal surface, in which case the bracket is put in a position which allows the tooth to be tied in and derotation commenced. Later the band must be removed and the bracket rewelded in the correct position. In the case of rotated teeth it is sometimes useful intentionally to place the bracket towards the mesial or distal surface of the tooth so that overcorrection of the rotation can be achieved more easily (*Fig.* 4.3A).

The level at which the brackets lie on the labial or buccal surfaces of the teeth is a matter of considerable importance. Vertical discrepancies in the level of the bracket channels will result in similar vertical discrepancies in tooth position unless compensating bends are made in the archwires throughout treatment.

The bracket channel should be 3·5–4 mm from the incisal edge of the upper central incisors. Once the bracket level has been determined for the central incisors the same measurement must be used to position premolar and canine brackets. The bracket channel on the upper lateral incisors must be approximately 1 mm closer to the incisal edge,

17

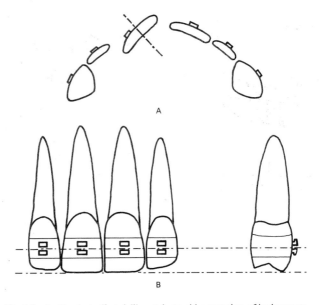

*Fig.* 4.3. A, Bracket offset deliberately to aid correction of incisor rotation. B, Bracket height on central and lateral incisors and second premolar.

so that at the completion of treatment the clinical crowns of the lateral incisors can remain slightly shorter than those of the central incisors (*Fig.* 4.3B).

### Molar Tubes

Various patterns of preformed weldable buccal attachments are available with either round or rectangular tubes.

Some preformed tubes are made with a slot which is formed between the distal end of the tube and the band surface for the attachment of elastics or tieback ligatures. A more advantageous position for the attachment of elastics is mesiobuccally, and preformed molar tubes with hooks in this position are available.

When extra-oral traction is to be applied to upper molars, preformed weldable double buccal tubes may be attached to the molar bands.

In order to simplify the fitting of the extra-oral arch, the extra-oral tube should lie occlusally and the archwire tube gingivally.

### Molar Tube Position

The buccal tubes on molar bands are placed parallel with the occlusal surface of the molar and parallel with the mesiodistal axis of the tooth.

18

When extra-oral traction is to be applied to a severely rotated upper molar, it may be necessary to angle the buccal tube away from the mesiodistal axis in order to facilitate insertion of the extra-oral arch. It is usually advantageous to place lower molar tubes near the gingival edge of the band so that the archwire is less liable to distortion by occlusal forces (*Fig. 4.4*).

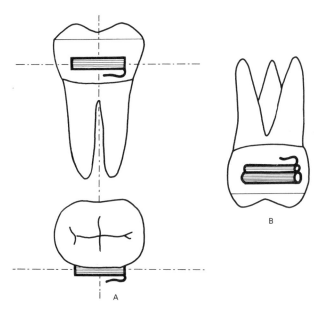

*Fig.* 4.4. A, Lower molar tube position. B, Double buccal tube on upper molar.

### Attachments

There is a variety of attachments which may be welded or soldered to bands and which provide additional points for attachment of elastics or tie ligatures (*Fig. 4.5*).

HOOKS: These are usually made from soft 0·7 mm stainless-steel wire, and soldered to the band. Preformed molar tubes with hooks are also available. Hooks on molar bands are usually placed mesiobuccally, gingivally to the molar tube. They are used for the attachment of intra- or intermaxillary traction elastics and for tieback ligatures. Hooks may also be placed mesiolingually for the attachment of elastics. Mesiolingual hooks are particularly useful for the uprighting of lower molars which have rolled lingually.

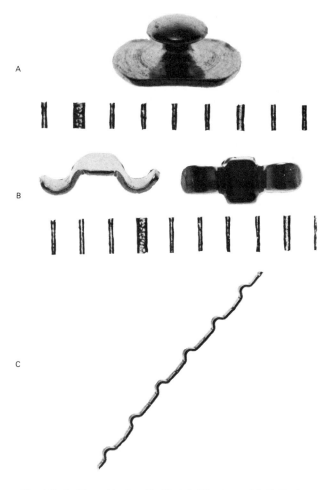

*Fig.* 4.5. A, Lingual button. B, Cleat (millimetre scale). C, Eyelets.

Hooks which are to be used for the attachment of cross elastics, when a crossbite is being corrected, are positioned vertically on the band.

All hooks, but particularly lingual hooks, must be positioned and designed in such a way as not to cause irritation to neighbouring soft tissues.

LINGUAL BUTTONS: Preformed lingual buttons may be used instead of lingual hooks on molars. They may also be fixed to premolar and canine bands for the attachment of elastic ligature, latex elastics, bracket elastics, or tie ligatures.

CLEATS AND EYELETS: These small preformed attachments are used for the attachment of tie ligatures, and are particularly useful for severely rotated or partially erupted teeth, when a bracket cannot be placed on the band in its correct position because of rotation or impaction. The tooth can be tied to the arch, and a bracket added at a later date when the tooth is nearer its correct position in the arch.

## CEMENTATION

Careful cementation of bands is vital to ensure successful results with fixed appliances, and to minimize the risk of decalcification of teeth. When the bands are being positioned, great care must be exercised to ensure that band angulation and bracket position are correct. For ease and accuracy of cementation there must be adequate tooth separation.

Some operators cement bands at the same visit as they are selected. It is then easy to remember exactly how a band seats on a particular tooth and which bands are difficult to place. Furthermore, the problem of band storage does not arise. The use of cement which has nearly set, will result in inadequately seated bands. The number of bands that can be placed satisfactorily with one mix of cement is limited. When cementing incisor bands particularly in a crowded lower arch it is wise to cement the canines and incisors with the same mix of cement. Even when incisors have been adequately separated the thickness of the band material can make the seating of bands difficult. To overcome this the bands must be seated progressively.

### The Teeth

Prior to cementation, the teeth which are to be banded must be thoroughly polished with prophylactic paste to remove plaque, then they must be dried and kept dry during cementation. An aspirator is very useful during band cementation. If cottonwool rolls are used to isolate the teeth they should be removed immediately before the bands are cemented, otherwise the cottonwool may easily become trapped under the gingival edge of the band. When the cement has set, any excess should be removed from the teeth and the bands. When bands are not selected and cemented at the same visit they must be carefully stored and labelled. The fit surface of the band must be clean and dry, and must be completely filled with cement before being seated on the tooth.

Edgewise brackets can be fitted with preformed bracket protectors which prevent the cement from entering the archwire channel or tie channel. Begg brackets and molar tubes can be protected by using ribbon wax, but care must be taken to ensure that the wax does not adhere to the fitting surface of the band.

*Cements*

There are two main types of cement for orthodontic use; zinc oxyphosphate and silicophosphate. The cement used depends largely upon operator preference, but the following points should be considered:

ZINC OXYPHOSPHATE: This is often mixed incorrectly. Ideally the slab must be cool and dry, and the powder incorporated into the liquid by

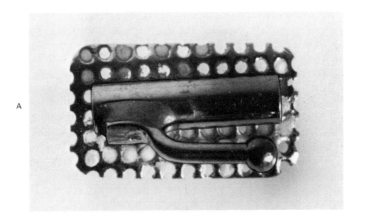

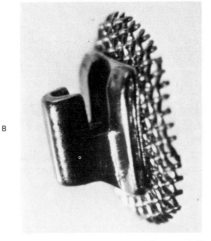

*Fig.* 4.6. A, A molar tube for direct bonding. B, A Begg bracket for direct bonding.

dividing it into five portions and incorporating a portion every 15 seconds. The common practice of mixing a very small quantity of powder into the liquid at the start, to delay the setting time, is not to be recommended for orthodontic use as it results in a weaker mix.

SILICOPHOSPHATE: The mixing of this cement is not as critical as that of zinc cements. It is mixed to a thicker consistency than zinc cements, and this makes band seating a little more difficult. It is very suitable for cementing a number of bands at one mix, as it gives a longer working time than zinc cements.

## DIRECT BONDING

Developments in the field of dental adhesives have made possible the bonding of attachments directly to the tooth surface. Brackets, molar tubes or lingual buttons (*Fig.* 4.6) may all be attached in this manner. The advantages of direct bonding are:

1. Separation of teeth is not necessary.

2. There is less danger of damage to the gingival tissues.

3. Direct bonding of attachments avoids the discomfort to the patient which is associated with banding.

4. There is no need to stock a large and expensive range of preformed bands.

5. Partially erupted teeth can have brackets or attachments directly bonded onto them.

6. Improvement in aesthetics.

7. At the completion of treatment, there is no residual space between the teeth, which normally arises following band removal as a

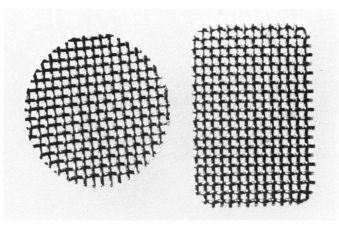

*Fig.* 4.7. Stainless-steel gauze for welding to brackets for direct bonding.

result of the thickness of the band material between the contact points.

Failure of direct bonding can occur at two sites, either the junction between the bonding material and the enamel, or at the junction between the bonding agent and the bracket. To improve the bond with the enamel, the teeth are acid etched, usually with phosphoric acid, which gives the enamel surface a microscopic porous structure which extends to a depth of 5–25 microns. The bond between the adhesive and stainless-steel is less satisfactory, and brackets have to be backed with stainless-steel gauze or perforated material (*Fig.* 4.7) to form a mechanical bond.

Plastic brackets are less conspicuous (*Fig.* 4.8) but their main disadvantage is that they are less rigid than stainless-steel brackets and may distort, or fracture, under the influence of occlusal forces generated by the archwire.

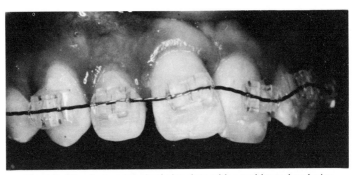

*Fig.* 4.8. Directly bonded plastic brackets with a multistrand archwire for initial incisor alignment.

*Adhesives*

A number of adhesive materials are available. The setting of the material is the result of chemical reaction or, in the case of some diacrylate resins, by means of ultraviolet light. It is obviously desirable to have a setting time long enough to enable the brackets to be positioned on the teeth accurately, but permitting the archwire to be tied in without delay.

Great care should be taken to follow the manufacturers' recommendations when using direct bonding systems.

### REFERENCES

Adams C. P. (1975) *The Design and Construction of Removable Appliances.* Bristol, Wright.
Beresford J. S. (1966) In: Walther D. P. (ed.), *Current Orthodontics.* Bristol, Wright, p. 320.

Gardiner J. H. and Aamodt A. C. (1968) *Trans. Br. Soc. Study Orthod.* **55,** 89.

Graber T. M. (1966) *Orthodontics.* Philadelphia, Saunders.

Houston W. J. B and Miller M. W. (1967) *Trans. Br. Soc. Study Orthod.* **54,** 120.

Reynolds I. R. (1975) *Br. J. Orthod.* **2,** 171.

Zachrisson B. U. (1977) *Am. J. Orthod.* **71,** 173.

CHAPTER 5

# ARCH FORM

The purpose of orthodontic treatment is not the reduction of all malocclusions to some 'norm' of occlusion. The diagnostic considerations which should determine the positions into which teeth are moved are not within the scope of this book. In describing arch form and the ultimate position into which the teeth should be moved, we have adopted a dogmatic approach based on the concept of stability of the lower labial segment (Mills, 1967). This is best followed whilst the operator gains experience in the use of fixed appliances. The overall arch form which is seen before treatment commences provides vital information about the positions into which teeth can be moved if they are to be stable following treatment. Since each successive archwire helps to determine the arch form at the end of treatment, archwire design must take into account the tooth movements to be undertaken, the original shape of the arch, and the final arch form intended. This chapter describes the principles which govern the overall archwire form.

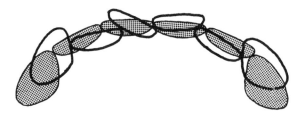

*Fig.* 5.1. Averaging of a crowded lower labial segment. The canines have been moved distally and the incisors aligned within the original curvature of the arch.

## THE LOWER ARCH

The labiolingual position of the lower incisor crowns is, in general, not stable if significantly altered by appliance mechanisms. The implication of this is that if space is created for alignment in a crowded lower arch by labial movement of the lower incisor crowns, crowding is likely to recur following appliance removal as the lower incisor crowns relapse towards their original labiolingual position.

Crowding in the lower incisor region will often be associated with a relative difference in the labiolingual position of the lower incisor crowns. Correction of this irregularity involves averaging their labiolingual positions to bring the lower incisors into alignment (*Fig. 5.1*). The space required for this movement is made available by distal movement of the lower canines. The anterior span of the lower archwire should thus form a smooth curve between the canines, the radius of curvature being related to the arch form before treatment.

The positions that the lower canines occupy are important, particularly in a buccolingual direction. If the intercanine width is 'overexpanded' in order to provide space for incisor alignment, the canines tend to relapse in a lingual direction following removal of the appliance. Every archwire should therefore be checked to ensure that it will not cause inadvertent increase in the intercanine width.

The buccolingual position of lower molars, unless they are being moved mesially or distally, is changed only when treating a molar crossbite. Care must be taken when placing archwires that they do not produce unwanted buccolingual movement of teeth in the buccal segments.

Buccal or lingual displacement of lower premolars is often seen; for example, lingual displacement of lower second premolars associated with crowding. Relief of crowding in that region will provide space for the movement of such teeth into a stable position in line with the other teeth in the buccal segment.

The buccal surfaces of 7654 | 4567 ideally lie in a straight line extending distally from the lower canines, except that the molar crowns are more bulbous than the premolar crowns. The buccal span of archwires should thus extend distally in a straight line from the lower canines. A bayonet bend (molar offset) may be incorporated in the archwire just in front of the molars in order to accommodate the bulbosity of the molar crowns.

The buccal spans of an archwire should diverge distally in order to accommodate the greater distance between lower molars as compared with that between lower first premolars.

## THE UPPER ARCH

Alteration of the labiolingual position of the upper incisor crowns is often required as part of orthodontic treatment, the incisor crowns being moved from one position of stability to another. If an increased overjet is to be completely reduced, the radius of curvature of the section of arc upon which the upper incisors will come to lie will be determined principally by the curvature of the lower labial segment.

Aesthetic considerations connected with the position of teeth in the upper labial segment are further satisfied by buccal offsets mesial to the upper canines, to allow these teeth to assume a more 'prominent' position relative to the incisors, and by small offsets mesial to each lateral incisor, to allow the labial surfaces of these teeth to lie in a slightly more palatal position than the labial surfaces of the central incisors (*Fig.* 5.2).

The factors which determine the buccolingual position of teeth in the upper buccal segments are similar to those which have been described for the lower buccal segments. The buccal span of archwire should be essentially straight, running distally from the canine, except for the molar offset. The buccal spans diverge distally.

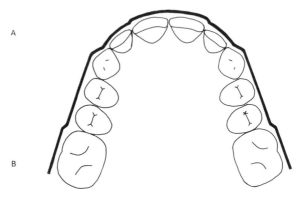

*Fig.* 5.2. Ideal arch form. A, Canine offsets. B, Molar offsets.

## ARCH SYMMETRY

Perfect bilateral symmetry of dental arches is probably rarely seen. In some patients, there is obvious bilateral asymmetry, associated with skeletal asymmetry, which cannot be permanently altered by orthodontic means. On the other hand, arches which are virtually symmetrical at the beginning of treament can be made asymmetric unless adequate attention is paid to archwire form. Such induced asymmetry is likely to relapse when the appliance is removed, and the resulting tooth movement may lead to a deterioration of the occlusion. Bilateral symmetry of archwires is checked by placing the archwire over millimetre-squared graph paper. Archwire correlation is assessed by comparing the upper and lower archwires.

## VERTICAL MOVEMENTS

Teeth which are vertically displaced in the arch may be moved by means of the archwire into vertical alignment with the other teeth. The general configuration of both upper and lower archwires is therefore 'flat' in the horizontal plane.

A particularly important vertical alteration in tooth position is 'depression' of lower incisors, which is described in Chapter 11.

## REFERENCES

Begg P. R. and Kesling P. C. (1977) *Orthodontic Theory and Technique*, 3rd
  ed. Philadelphia, Saunders, chapter 2.
Mills J. R. E. (1967) *Trans. Br. Soc. Study Orthod.* **54,** 11.
Tweed C. H. (1966) *Clinical Orthodontics,* vol. 1. St. Louis, Mosby.

# CHAPTER 6

# BRACKETS AND ARCHWIRES

Fixed-appliance mechanisms depend upon being able to attach an archwire to groups of teeth. Brackets are rigidly fixed to the teeth, and the precise interrelation of bracket and archwire is thus of prime importance in determining the action of the appliance.

## BRACKET AND ARCHWIRE COMBINATIONS

In order to illustrate the implications of the relationship between brackets and archwire, three combinations will be described.

### 1. *Edgewise Brackets and Rectangular Archwire*

The archwire and brackets are precision products and the wire fits accurately into the bracket, with the result that the tooth is thus 'locked' on to the archwire in all planes (*Fig.* 6.1A). The system has obvious advantages in providing the possibility of precise control of tooth position. It also has disadvantages. The relationship of bracket and archwire demands precise archwire fabrication and bracket positioning. Unless the archwire is very carefully adjusted, unwanted activations will be introduced. The relative inflexibility of the rectangular archwire means that, unless care is taken, excessive forces are applied to the teeth. Accurate tooth positioning, often involving apical movement, requires a considerable amount of anchorage and usually necessitates the use of extra-oral traction.

### 2. *Edgewise Brackets and Round-wire Arch*

This combination differs from the previous example in that the bracket, and hence the tooth, is free to rotate in one plane, as the archwire does not fit tightly into the bracket channel (*Fig.* 6.1B). The mesiodistal width of the bracket allows for a tooth to be rotated or uprighted. Because of the freedom of the tooth to rotate on the archwire, labial or lingual movement of incisor roots is not possible unless 'two-point contact' is established by modification of the archwire or the addition of accessory arches.

Edgewise brackets are available in a range of mesiodistal widths. Siamese brackets are specifically designed to give a large mesiodistal width, thus facilitating rotation and uprighting. The width of the bracket, however, restricts the tipping of teeth *along* the archwire.

### 3. Begg Brackets and Round-wire Arch

The Begg bracket has minimal mesiodistal width, and the archwire is a loose fit in the bracket. As a result the teeth are free to tip along and around the archwire. Accessory springs must be used to produce apical movement, and because of the minimal mesiodistal width of the bracket, springs or elastics are sometimes necessary to produce rotation of teeth (*Fig.* 6.1C).

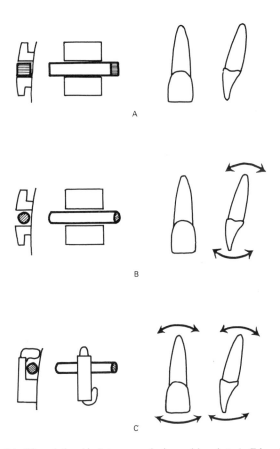

*Fig.* 6.1. The relationship between archwire and bracket. A, Edgewise bracket and rectangular archwire. Tooth movement is controlled in all planes. B, Edgewise bracket and round archwire. The tooth can rotate around the archwire. C, Begg bracket and round archwire. The tooth can rotate around the archwire and tip along the archwire.

## PROPERTIES OF ORTHODONTIC WIRES

When a load is applied to a wire, the wire will deform. As the load is increased and the stress (force per unit cross-sectional area) on the wire rises, the wire deforms elastically until the *elastic limit* is reached. The amount of deformation produced is directly proportional to the load applied, and a wire which has been deformed elastically will return to its initial shape if the load is removed.

As the wire is progressively stressed beyond its elastic limit, further deformation will occur, but now the wire will take on a permanent 'set', and will not return to its initial shape if the load is removed. Deformation accompanied by permanent bending is referred to as plastic deformation. Yet further stressing will eventually result in breakage of the wire (*Fig.* 6.2).

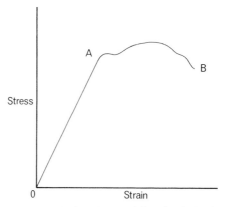

*Fig.* 6.2. Load deflection characteristics of orthodontic wire. A, Elastic limit. B, Breaking point. O–A represents elastic deformation. A–B represents plastic deformation.

The load deflection characteristics of a wire are of considerable significance to the orthodontist. If the wire has to be formed before being tied in, it has to be plastically deformed without reaching its breaking point. When tied into the brackets its elastic deformation characteristics may be used to produce tooth movement.

The behaviour of a formed archwire is related to its diameter, its physical properties, and to the length of archwire between brackets on adjacent teeth.

### The Influence of Wire Diameter

Consider two wires of the same length, composition and manufacture, one having a diameter of 0·3 mm and the other a diameter of 0·6 mm (*Fig.* 6.3).

32

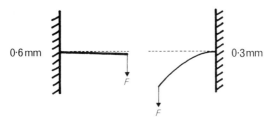

*Fig.* 6.3. Load deflection characteristics of two wires of different diameters, but the same length. The 0·30 mm diameter wire must be deflected 16 times as far as the 0·60 mm diameter wire to apply the same force.

In order to apply a given force, the thinner wire must be deflected 16 times as far as the thicker wire (assuming elastic deformation).

This can be expressed in the formula $d \propto 1/r^4$, where $d$ represents deflection and $r$ the radius of the wire.

The diameter of the wire thus has a major influence upon its elastic properties. The most commonly used sizes of high tensile round wire range from 0·3 mm to 0·55 mm in 0·05 mm increments. The smaller diameters are used when maximum flexibility is required, because these wires can be deformed elastically over relatively large distances without applying excessive forces or becoming plastically deformed. Thus a plain (that is, without loops) small diameter archwire may be used to produce initial alignment when there is considerable tooth displacement.

The larger diameters of archwire are used when rigidity is desirable, and the intermediate sizes are used as required in order to match the qualities of the archwire to the tooth displacement.

Multistrand wires are manufactured by braiding together three fine high tensile stainless-steel wires. They are more flexible than a single strand wire of the same overall diameter. Full engagement of the archwire in the bracket can be obtained at an early stage, and permanent archwire deformation under masticatory forces is minimized. The difficulty with such wire is that its flexibility becomes inconvenient in those parts of its length where rigidity is required. This usually applies to the teeth acting as anchorage, generally the molars. The archwire is too flexible to prevent unwanted movement of molars, especially if elastic inter- or intramaxillary traction (*see* p. 46) is applied. Furthermore, the archwire is too flexible to enable lower incisors to be 'depressed'. These very flexible archwires find their main application at an early stage of treatment, to produce rapid initial correction of occlusal, labiolingual, and rotational displacements (*Fig.* 6.4).

In the Johnson twin-wire arch two small diameter wires are used to

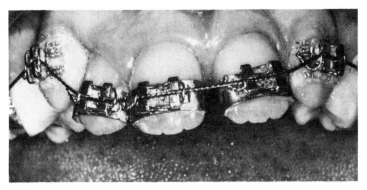

*Fig.* 6.4. A multistrand archwire to bring 3|3 occlusally.

provide flexibility, and they are supported in the buccal segments, where more rigidity is required, by enclosing them in end tubes (*Fig.* 6.5). The superior flexibility and ease of application of multistrand wires have to a large extent led to the supplanting of the Johnson twin-wire arch (*see* p. 148).

Rectangular wires are relatively rigid and when edgewise brackets are used, much of the alignment is achieved using more flexible, round wires. Rectangular wires are sometimes only used in the final stages of treatment, when the precision of the archwire–bracket combination enables great accuracy in tooth positioning to be achieved. When rectangular wires are used, some operators increase the flexibility of particular sections of archwire by selective electrolytic reduction.

### The Physical Properties of the Wire

A number of austenitic stainless-steel archwire materials are available for orthodontic use. They vary in their composition, manufacture, and

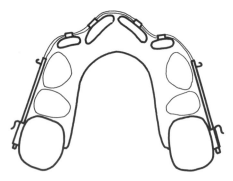

*Fig.* 6.5. Johnson twin-wire arch.

elastic properties. Some wires are produced in coils, others in straight lengths. The choice of a particular product rests largely with the operator. Wires supplied with the same nominal diameter in fact vary in this dimension. In addition, the elastic properties of a wire are altered by clinical forming. The elastic limit of a wire made from austenitic stainless-steel and its range of elastic deformation is increased during manufacture by alternate cycles of cold working and heating to relieve stress. 'Heat-treated' or 'high tensile' stainless-steel wire is the material most commonly used for the construction of round archwires.

Elgiloy wire is a chromium–nickel–cobalt alloy which can be used for the construction of archwires. It is formed by plastic deformation in its 'soft' state, but unlike stainless-steel it can then be 'hardened', in order to improve its elastic properties, by heating alone.

Formed archwires made from stainless-steel can be heat-treated to relieve internal stress, so making the archwire more resistant to fracture. Some orthodontic welders have terminals designed to enable a current to be passed through an archwire, the electrical resistance of which then causes its temperature to rise. It is not possible by this method to achieve even heating when the archwire incorporates bends and loops, and there is a danger of annealing the wire. An alternative method of heating is to use an oven, but this is time consuming. In view of the quality of stainless-steel archwire materials now available, it is doubtful if the benefits of heat-treating formed stainless-steel round archwires justify the effort.

### The Influence of Wire Length

Consider two wires of the same diameter, composition, and manufacture, each supported between two points. The deflection required to produce a given force in the middle of the span will depend upon the distance between the supports (*Fig. 6.6*).

If the distance between the supports is doubled then the deflection required to produce a given force is increased by a factor of eight. This fact is expressed in the formula $d \propto l^3$, where $d$ represents deflection and $l$ the distance between the supports.

The length of archwire in a span is therefore of considerable importance, and can be increased by the incorporation of loops (*Fig. 6.7*).

## ARCHWIRE DESIGN

In its relationship to individual teeth in an arch, the requirements of an archwire vary. In some areas the archwire is being deformed elastically to produce tooth movement, so flexibility is required in order that plastic deformation does not occur. At the same time, sufficient force

35

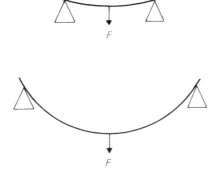

*Fig.* 6.6. Load deflection characteristics of two wires of the same diameter between supports. In the lower diagram the distance between the supports is twice that in the upper diagram. The deflection required to produce a given force is increased by a factor of eight if the distance between the supports is doubled.

to initiate tooth movement must be generated, and excessive forces avoided.

In other areas the function of the archwire is to prevent unwanted tooth movement and perhaps to support accessories, and in these areas rigidity is required.

It is difficult to combine the properties of flexibility and rigidity in a single archwire, and a degree of compromise usually has to be accepted. For clarification of the way in which archwires function, we have divided them into two categories:

1. Active archwires: these are designed in such a way that tooth-moving forces are generated by attaching the archwire to the teeth.

2. Base archwires: these do not themselves produce movement of teeth to which they are attached; they act as a support for accessories, which produce tooth movement.

In practice these types of archwire are not mutually exclusive, but the principles involved are entirely different, and they will now be described in greater detail as separate entities.

### Active Archwires

These archwires are designed in such a way that, when teeth are ligated to them, the archwire is distorted from its passive form so that forces are applied to the teeth.

Teeth attached to such an archwire thus move 'with the archwire' as it reverts to its passive state. Because the teeth move with the archwire rather than along the archwire, the maximum potential of the

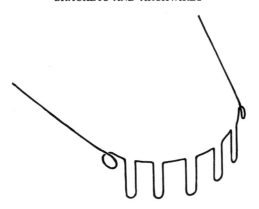

*Fig*. 6.7. A multilooped archwire for the alignment of a crowded lower labial segment. The circle hooks are for the attachment of elastic traction.

relationship between brackets and archwire is realized, particularly if full engagement of the archwire in the brackets is maintained. When using brackets of appreciable mesiodistal width, maximum control is realized by firmly attaching the archwire to the bracket and so achieving tooth movement by allowing the tooth and the segment of archwire in the bracket to move together as a unit.

Active archwires must be sufficiently flexible to produce significant tooth movement without applying excessive forces or becoming plastically deformed.

*Design of Active Archwires*

The flexibility of an archwire span between neighbouring brackets is influenced by the design of the span, the diameter and composition of the wire, and the type of bracket used. *Fig*. 6.8 illustrates that the span of archwire between Begg brackets is larger than between edgewise brackets when a plain archwire is used.

The significance of this aspect of bracket–archwire relationship is that, particularly when wide brackets are used for correcting appreciable tooth displacement, inter-bracket archwire flexibility must be obtained by reducing archwire diameter or by lengthening the span, if full bracket engagement is to be achieved without permanent archwire deformation. The inter-bracket span of archwire can be lengthened by the incorporation of loops (*see below*).

The width of the brackets has a further important influence upon the characteristics of a span. *Fig*. 6.9 illustrates the alignment of a tooth using Begg or edgewise brackets.

37

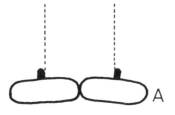

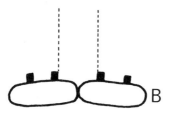

*Fig.* 6.8. Inter-bracket distance with (A) Begg brackets, and (B) edgewise brackets.

It should be noticed that even in this relatively simple instance there may be movement induced in teeth at some distance from the site of intended activation. The rigidity of the inter-bracket spans is considerably increased if the archwire is fully engaged in wide (Siamese edgewise) brackets.

Frictional forces also play a part in determining the action of an elastically deformed span, and once again the design of bracket is of significance. *Fig.* 6.10 illustrates the alignment of a single tooth using either Begg or edgewise brackets. There is just sufficient space to accommodate the displaced tooth.

If the displaced tooth is to move into alignment between the other teeth either the bracket points a and b must separate, or the archwire must slide through the brackets. *Fig.* 6.10A illustrates the situation where Siamese edgewise brackets have been used. Frictional forces have prevented movement of the archwire through the bracket channels, and points a and b have separated. Clinically, separation of

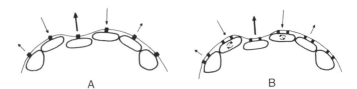

*Fig.* 6.9. Labial movement of a lower incisor using plain round archwire with (A) Begg brackets, and (B) edgewise brackets.

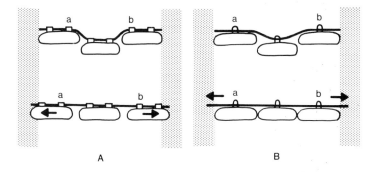

*Fig.* 6.10. The effect of frictional forces when using (A) edgewise brackets and (B) Begg brackets.

points a and b may be demonstrated by movement of teeth along the arch or by proclination onto an arc of larger diameter (*see* for example, incisor proclination, Chapter 10). *Fig.* 6.10B illustrates the situation where Begg brackets have been used. The narrowness of the bracket, and the loose fit of the archwire in the bracket channel, has allowed the archwire to move through the brackets. Conditions elsewhere in the arch have been ignored in order to illustrate the possible implications of friction (bracket binding). In practice the situation is likely to be further complicated by restriction of tooth or archwire movement elsewhere in the arch, and if crowding is present part of the applied force will be distributed through inter-dental contact points.

*Multilooped Archwires*

The inter-bracket span of archwire can be increased in length by the incorporation of loops. In this way it is possible to construct an archwire of sufficient diameter (for example, 0·4 mm) to resist unwanted movement in one area, yet flexible enough to produce tooth movement in another.

The flexibility of plain archwires is similar in both horizontal and vertical displacement. Small diameter plain archwires are therefore useful in the early stages of treatment. Their principal drawback is that they are not rigid enough to resist unwanted movement. Looped archwires are more difficult to construct, but can be designed in such a way as to introduce maximum flexibility in areas of maximum tooth displacement.

The flexibility of looped sections of archwire is, unlike plain sections, not equal in both horizontal and vertical planes. Vertical loops are most useful in increasing the flexibility of a span of archwire in a

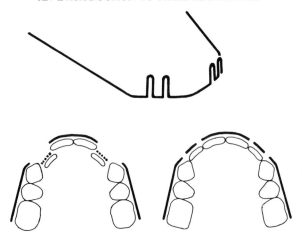

*Fig.* 6.11. Active archwire, 0·40 mm diameter, with vertical loops to procline 2 2. A, Archwire in place; the broken line shows position when the archwire is tied into the brackets on 2|2. B, Completion of tooth movement.

buccolingual direction (*Fig.* 6.11). *Fig.* 6.12 illustrates that the flexibility of a span in a buccolingual direction is increased by lengthening and widening the vertical loops, although local conditions will obviously set limits to these dimensions.

In practice vertical loops extend into the sulcus 5–6 mm from the level of the archwire. They must not impinge on the gingiva or protrude into the cheek or lip.

Vertical loops are much less flexible in vertical displacement than in horizontal displacement. *Fig.* 6.13 illustrates a looped span which is designed to provide flexibility in vertical displacement.

Careful planning and activation of vertical loops will also enable limited mesiodistal movement of teeth to be achieved. An archwire with a vertically looped labial section is particularly useful in dealing with a crowded lower incisor region, as labiolingual, rotational, and mesiodistal movement of the incisors can be effected simultaneously (*see* Chapter 10).

The mechanics of vertically looped archwires is complex, and may present problems of overbite reduction and anchorage control. They should be discarded in favour of plain archwires, which are easier to control, when tooth displacement does not demand maximum archwire flexibility.

In summary, the alignment of severe displacements may be commenced with small (0·30 mm, 0·35 mm) diameter plain round wires, changing to medium (0·40 mm, 0·45 mm) diameter round multi-

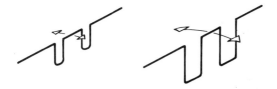

Fig. 6.12. Flexibility of a span of archwire in a buccolingual direction is increased by lengthening and widening the vertical loops.

looped archwires, and finishing with plain round archwires (0·45 mm–0·5 mm). When edgewise brackets are used, rectangular archwires may be used after initial alignment with plain and multi-looped round archwires.

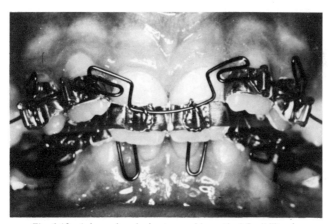

Fig. 6.13. A looped archwire to provide vertical flexibility.

### Base Archwires

These archwires are plain, often thicker than active archwires, and as a result are more rigid. They support tooth-moving accessories, such as coil springs, uprighting springs, and elastics.

In addition to supporting accessories, base archwires influence the direction in which the teeth move. The agents producing the tooth movement are the accessories, and the teeth move relative to the archwire, so that the system depends upon there being a loose fit of the archwire in the brackets. The full potential of the relationship between brackets and archwire for controlling movement is therefore not realized.

An accessory can be used to move a tooth along a base archwire. If a bracket of appreciable mesiodistal width is used and the tooth tips

41

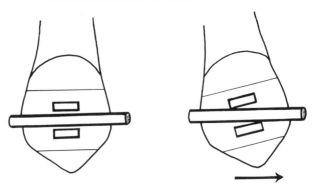

*Fig.* 6.14. When a tooth is moved along an archwire and becomes tipped, binding occurs between the bracket and archwire.

under the influence of the applied force, the bracket will bind on the archwire and further tipping will be prevented (*Fig.* 6.14). As soon as a tooth binds on an archwire, part of the force intended to move that tooth will be transmitted through the archwire to other teeth. The magnitude of the force dissipated in this manner is impossible to measure and its effects are unpredictable.

### *Accessories*

The accessories which are used in conjunction with base archwires to produce tooth movements are elastics, whips and uprighting springs, and coil springs.

### *Elastics*

Elastic is available in several forms for orthodontic use. Commercially produced latex elastic loops are used for applying inter- or intra-maxillary traction, and they are available in various sizes. They are manufactured to close tolerances, and bands of a given size have nearly identical load/deflection characteristics. The force delivered by latex loops decreases as the material remains in the mouth, due to absorption of water from the saliva.

Natural rubber bands are not of standard size, and they absorb more water from the saliva than do latex elastics; they are therefore not satisfactory as the force applied by them cannot be carefully controlled.

Elastics should normally be worn full time, and even when breakage does not occur latex loops should ideally be replaced daily. One of the disadvantages of elastics is that they depend upon the co-operation of the patient, who must be able to insert them and must be aware of the necessity of full-time wear. When choosing the appropriate-sized elastic, a tension gauge should be used to measure the force applied.

Commercially produced elastic loops, chains, and threads are manufactured from a synthetic elastic material. Small single loops (bracket elastics) are available for maintaining the engagement of an archwire in edgewise brackets. The chain bracket elastics may be used for mesiodistal tooth movement along an archwire or for rotation of a tooth. They are not as elastic as latex.

Elastic ligature, which is available in reels, is mainly used for closing spaces and producing rotation of teeth (*Fig.* 6.15). It has the

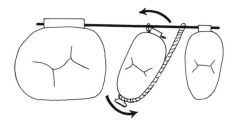

Fig. 6.15. Elastic ligature to derotate a premolar.

disadvantage of being difficult for the patient to keep clean, and in certain situations is liable to breakage. It should be renewed at each appointment.

## *Whips and Uprighting Springs*

These are accessory springs which are used to align individual teeth. Uprighting springs produce mesiodistal tipping, and whip springs, or rotation springs, produce rotation of a tooth about its long axis. When Begg brackets are used these accessory springs are essential for producing apical movement in a mesiodistal direction. By contrast, accessory springs are not commonly employed with edgewise brackets, although certain edgewise brackets are made with a vertical channel to accommodate uprighting springs (e.g. Broussard).

UPRIGHTING SPRINGS: These are used in conjunction with Begg brackets to produce apical movement in a mesiodistal direction. They are made from 0·30 mm or 0·35 mm diameter high tensile stainless-steel wire. One end is accommodated in the vertical channel of the bracket and the other is engaged on the archwire (*Fig.* 6.17).

When a tooth is being uprighted the reciprocal forces are such that the crown will tend to move in the opposite direction to the root apex and the tooth will tend to be extruded. In order to prevent these unwanted movements the tooth must be ligated to the archwire and tied back to an adjacent tooth.

**ROTATION SPRINGS OR WHIPS:** These springs are used to produce rotation of an individual tooth around its long axis.

When a Begg bracket is used the rotation spring engages the vertical channel of the bracket, and the emerging end is bent at right angles to the labial or buccal surface to establish a two-point contact on the tooth (*Fig.* 6.16).

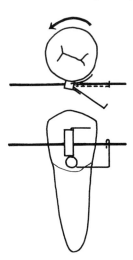

*Fig.* 6.16. Accessory spring used with Begg bracket to produce rotation.

With an edgewise bracket a whip spring does not incorporate a coil (*Fig.* 6.17E). The archwire at the point of engagement of the whip is liable to distortion, and therefore it is advisable to use a base archwire of at least 0·45 mm in order to reduce the possibility of unwanted tooth movement. The tooth to be moved must be ligated to the archwire.

With edgewise brackets the indication for the use of rotation whips is when a tooth is relatively severely rotated in an otherwise well-aligned arch.

*Coil Springs*

Coil springs are wound from hard stainless-steel wire. The coil spring is made to be expanded when passive—it is intended to push rather than pull. Coil springs find their main application in opening space. The spring is compressed between the brackets of the teeth to be separated (*Fig.* 6.18).

Coil springs can be used for mesial or distal movement of teeth by compressing the coil against the bracket of the tooth to be moved either by a tie-back ligature or an archwire stop. The coil spring is free to move along the archwires as the tooth moves, but bracket binding may occur as the tooth tips. The most useful sizes are 0·15 mm wire

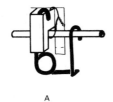

A

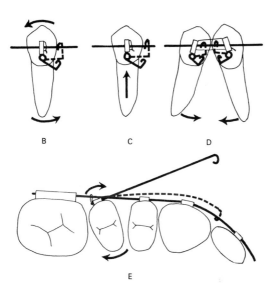

B           C           D

E

*Fig.* 6.17. Whips and uprighting springs. A, B, C, D, Begg uprighting springs. B, The effect of an uprighting spring is to move the crown and root in opposite directions. C, An uprighting spring imparts a vertical component of force to the tooth concerned. D, Crowns of $\overline{53|}$ tied together during uprighting. E, Whip to derotate a premolar. The premolar must be tied into the archwire to prevent it from being moved palatally.

wound on 0·7 mm, or 0·8 mm diameter wire. Coil springs have largely been replaced by elastic ligatures following the development of a satisfactory ligature material.

## INTRA-ORAL FORCES

Tooth-moving forces are generated in a number of ways: by elastic deformation of an archwire, by the use of accessory springs or coils,

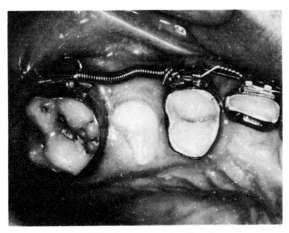

*Fig.* 6.18. A compressed coil spring.

or by the use of elastic components. Any tooth movement in an arch may have an effect upon the other teeth attached to the archwire. Elastic loops enable teeth in one arch to be moved by using teeth in the opposing arch as a site from which the force is delivered, the teeth in the opposing arch forming the anchorage unit.

### *Intramaxillary Traction*

This is the term used to describe forces applied either in the upper or lower arches, and its action is to close spaces and shorten the arch length. It is applied either by the activation of closing loops, or by elastic traction. When elastic loops are used, these are usually hooked over buccal hooks on molars and onto archwire hooks.

### *Archwire Hooks*

These are bent into the archwire, usually mesial to the canines, and may be used for the attachment of elastics or tie ligatures. They must be large enough to enable the patient to apply the elastic easily, but as unobtrusive as possible in order to minimize the chance of trauma to neighbouring soft tissues.

The circle hook and the Begg hook may lie horizontally or vertically according to local conditions (*Fig.* 6.19A and B).

The Begg hook is useful in that the right-angle bend at its distal end forms a stop which can then bear directly upon the mesial aspect of the canine bracket, so transferring a distally directed force positively to the canine.

46

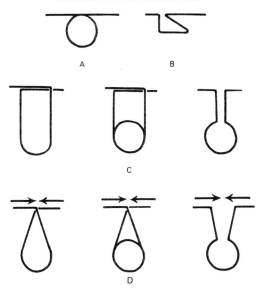

*Fig.* 6.19. A, Circle hook. B, Begg hook. C, Closing loops. D, Closing loops when activated.

## Closing and Opening Loops

An archwire can be made flexible in its length by the incorporation of vertical loops. Where a greater degree of flexibility is required a reverse loop which includes a helix can be used (*Fig.* 6.19C).

Closing loops are activated by pulling the archwire through the molar tube and turning the end down hard at the distal end of the molar tube. Alternatively, a traction hook can be bent up distal to the closing loops and used for the attachment of a tie-back ligature. This makes the archwire easier to remove and re-insert through the molar tubes if it has to be taken out for adjustment.

Vertical loops can also be constructed to increase the distance between two teeth (opening loops). The archwire must be inserted in the active state and the vertical arms of the opening loops are compressed between the brackets on the relevant teeth before the archwire is tied in.

### Intermaxillary Traction

This is a method of using one arch as anchorage for tooth movements in the other arch. The force is supplied by elastic loops connected between the two arches.

The effect of intermaxillary traction, like intramaxillary traction,

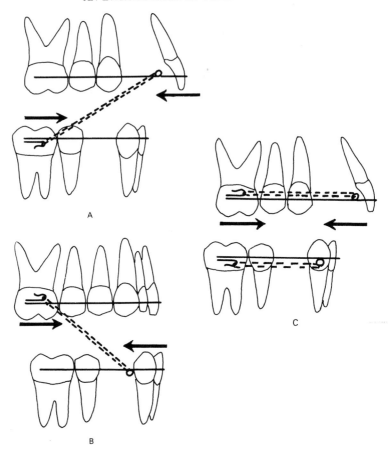

*Fig.* 6.20. Inter- and intramaxillary traction. A, Class II intermaxillary traction. B, Class III intermaxillary traction. C, Intramaxillary traction. This can be used in either the mandibular or maxillary arch.

depends upon the site of application of the force, the resistance of teeth to movement and the number of teeth to be moved.

'Class II traction' is the term used when the traction is from the front of the maxillary arch to the back of the mandibular arch and is used in the main for treatment of Class II malocclusions. Depending upon the arrangement of the upper archwire, Class II traction can provide a distal force to the whole upper arch and prevent forward movement of upper buccal segments, or it may be used to reduce an overjet. The reaction in the lower arch is to bring the lower buccal segments forwards, closing lower extraction spaces (*Fig.* 6.20A).

Class III traction is taken from the lower canine region to the distal aspect of the upper arch (*Fig.* 6.20B). The design of the lower archwire will determine whether the traction will apply a retroclining force to the lower incisors or a distal force to the lower buccal segments. In the upper arch it will move the first molars forwards, and this can be used to procline the upper incisors or to close spaces. As a general rule Class III traction is used in the treatment of Class III cases.

Intermaxillary traction is applied by means of elastics, and forces of 60–100 g are used on either side. The elastics are worn full time, including when eating, to obtain the maximum effect.

The elastics are attached to hooks or buttons on molar bands and to archwire hooks in the opposing arch.

Intramaxillary traction is commonly used in conjunction with intermaxillary traction. However, in many cases intra-oral anchorage is insufficient to carry out the desired tooth movements, in which case extra-oral anchorage is required to supplement intra-oral anchorage (*see* Chapter 8).

The use of intra- and extra-oral forces in anchorage control is discussed in more detail in Chapter 13.

## ARCH PLACEMENT

*Edgewise Brackets*

The archwire is tied into edgewise brackets, using either stainless-steel ligatures, or bracket elastics (*Fig.* 6.21).

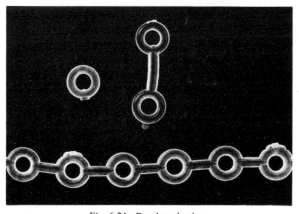

*Fig.* 6.21. Bracket elastics.

49

Stainless-steel ligatures are available preformed in a range of thickness, but 0·25 mm or 0·30 mm are commonly used. When tying in it is best to ligate those parts of the archwire that lie fully in the brackets first. The remaining brackets are then tied in, but care must be taken not to apply too much force, as this might produce permanent archwire deformation, or excessive forces on a particular tooth.

Where a tooth is rotated, and it is not possible to engage the archwire fully, the ligature is passed over the archwire at a single point only. The side of the bracket that is most displaced from the archwire is tied in, leaving the other side untied. This reduces friction and allows correction of the rotation to take place.

Bracket elastics may be used when the archwire lies in the bracket; they will not produce full bracket engagement where the archwire lies at some distance from the bracket. Linked bracket elastics may be used when space closure is required.

Positive and rapid location of the archwire in the bracket channel is best achieved using ligature locking pliers (*Fig.* 6.22).

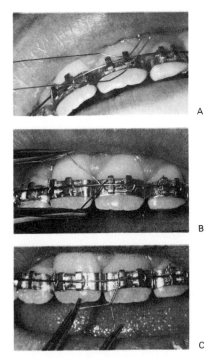

A

B

C

*Fig.* 6.22. Archwire ligation. A, A preformed ligature is placed over the archwire. B, The ligature is tightened with ligature locking pliers. C, The ligature is twisted, cut, and the end tucked under the archwire.

## Begg Brackets

When Begg brackets are being used the archwire is held in the bracket slot with a brass locking pin. When the archwire lies at a considerable distance from the bracket and full engagement would produce an excessive force, the archwire is loosely attached to the bracket with a stainless-steel ligature (*see Fig.* 6.13).

When a multilooped archwire is being placed it is best to attach the teeth which are not displaced from the archwire first, and then the teeth which are displaced. In this way the force applied to the teeth being aligned can be assessed as the archwire is tied in.

When tied in, no part of the archwire should press against the gingivae. The distal ends of the archwire must be adjusted so as not to traumatize the mucous membrane. Ligatures and hooks should be as unobtrusive as possible.

## REFERENCES

Begg P. R. and Kesling P. C. (1977) *Orthodontic Theory and Technique,* 3rd ed. Philadelphia, Saunders, Chapter 6.

Halden J. R. (1966) In: Walther, D. P. (ed.), *Current Orthodontics.* Bristol, Wright, p. 362.

Stephens C. D. and Waters N. E. (1971) *Dent. Pract. Dent. Rec.* **22,** 2.

Stephens C. D., Houston W. J. B. and Waters N. E. (1971) *Dent. Pract. Dent. Rec.* **22,** 147.

Tweed C. H. (1966) *Clinical Orthodontics.* St Louis, Mosby.

Waters N. E., Houston W. J. B. and Stephens C. D. (1976) *Br. J. Orthod.* **3,** 217.

CHAPTER 7

# PALATAL AND LINGUAL ARCHES

Palatal and lingual arches are relatively rigid arches fixed to molar bands. They have a variety of uses:

1. Space maintenance.
2. Anchorage.
3. Control of intermolar distance.
4. Attachment of auxiliaries.
5. Rotation of molars.
6. Proclination of lower incisors.
7. Distal movement of lower molars.

Of these, the first is the most important.

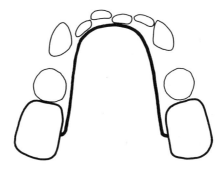

*Fig.* 7.1. Lingual arch used as a space maintainer. The arch is soldered to 6|6 bands and just touches the lingually placed incisors but must be kept clear of 3|3 to allow these teeth to move distally.

## SPACE MAINTENANCE

The extraction of teeth is often carried out as part of orthodontic treatment in order to relieve crowding. Space maintainers can be used to prevent spontaneous forward movement of buccal teeth following extractions in order that the extraction space is available for the alignment of anterior teeth (*Fig.* 7.1). Space maintainers are also used to retain space for unerupted or partially erupted teeth.

Palatal and lingual arches act as space maintainers because they: (1) maintain anteroposterior arch length; (2) maintain intermolar width; (3) prevent mesial tipping of molars; and (4) prevent molar rotation.

## Maintenance of Anteroposterior Arch Length

Palatal and lingual arches restrict forward movement of molars to which they are attached because the anterior section of the arch rests in contact with either the palatal mucosa or the lingual surfaces of the lower incisors. If, despite the arch, the molars move mesially, a palatal arch may become embedded in the palatal mucosa anteriorly, or a lingual arch may produce lower incisor proclination.

## Maintenance of Intermolar Width

Each dental arch converges towards the front of the mouth. Therefore, if a molar is to move anteriorly, it must also move towards the midline at the same time. Conversely, when molars are being moved distally, they must also be moved buccally. The rigidity of palatal and lingual arches maintains intermolar width, and thus prevents or minimizes forward movement of the molars.

## Prevention of Molar Tipping

When molars move forward spontaneously they are liable to tip mesially. Palatal and lingual arches 'lock' the molars together so that, if they do move forward, they must tip mesially by an identical amount. This in itself discourages forward movement. In addition, mesial tipping is restricted by virtue of the contact between the anterior section of the arch and the palatal mucosa or lower incisors. If, however, the molars do tip forwards when a palatal or lingual arch is in place, the anterior section of the arch will tend to move upwards in the upper arch and downwards in the lower. This will be demonstrated in the upper arch by the embedding of the palatal arch in the palatal mucosa, and in the lower arch by proclination of the incisors. The addition of an acrylic 'button' to the anterior section of a palatal arch has been found to be useful in that it dissipates the forces produced by molar movement over a greater surface area of the palate and therefore helps to restrict forward movement.

## Prevention of Molar Rotation

When molars, particularly upper molars, move forward spontaneously they are liable to rotate mesiopalatally. The rigidity of a palatal arch restricts this rotation.

When using a palatal or lingual arch for space maintenance, the arch should be soldered to the bands in order to make the appliance as rigid as possible.

In practice the indications for the use of space maintainers are limited for the following reasons:

1. They may be required over an extended period. The prolonged use of any appliance is to be avoided, if possible, because of the

possibility of damage to the teeth or gingivae. In addition, the patient's co-operation may fail if treatment extends over a long period.

2. In most cases where extractions are carried out to relieve crowding, the malocclusion can be more rapidly treated if active tooth movement is started relatively soon after the extractions are completed. Furthermore, controlled movement of buccal teeth is often desirable during the treatment of the malocclusion.

## Anchorage

As described above, the rigidity of palatal and lingual arches restricts movement of the molars. Molars to which these arches are attached will thus offer greater resistance to the forward movement which is liable to occur during canine and premolar retraction and incisor alignment.

Palatal and lingual arches can be used in conjunction with multi-band appliances to improve molar anchorage, but it must be remembered that they do not absolutely prevent forward movement of the molars. The molars may still move under the influence of forces applied by the rest of the appliance, and the palatal or lingual arch will then not lie in the intended position and may become a hindrance. Palatal and lingual arches are used to increase molar anchorage when sectional buccal arches are employed, for instance to produce canine retraction.

## Control of Intermolar Distance

Palatal or lingual arches can be used to maintain an intermolar 'expansion' previously obtained by using a removable appliance, or to

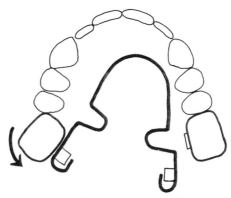

*Fig.* 7.2. Palatal arch used for molar rotation. The reaction to this movement is a distal force on the molar on the opposite side of the arch.

increase or decrease intermolar distance. An appreciable force is required to change the intermolar distance, and the arches need to be activated a total of 5–8 mm across the molars. When moving molars buccally or lingually it is preferable to use a removable arch, which can be detached from the bands for reactivation.

## Attachment of Auxiliaries

In the labiolingual technique, palatal and lingual arches are used for the attachment of auxiliary springs, which produce movement of teeth principally by tipping. Such appliances are sometimes useful for the attachment of palatal springs to align palatally displaced upper canines, or for the uprighting of lingually displaced second premolars.

## Rotation of Molars

Palatal and lingual arches can be activated to produce molar rotation. *Fig.* 7.2 demonstrates the activation of a palatal arch to rotate a molar mesiobuccally. Removable arches are used in order that they can be detached from the bands for reactivation. Because of their inflexibility care must be taken not to overactivate the arches.

## Proclination of Lower Incisors

Occasionally it is necessary to procline the lower incisors. For this movement a lingual arch incorporating U-loops lying just in front of the molar-band attachments can be used. The arch is activated by expansion of the U-loops so that the anterior section presses against the lingual surfaces of the lower incisors. Alternatively, the arch can be used to support a Friel spring for proclination of the incisors.

## Distal Movement of Lower Molars

Occasionally, where there is only very mild crowding of the lower arch, it may be decided to move the lower molars distally. A lower lingual arch may be used as described above, with activated U-loops to move the lower molars distally. The likelihood of proclining the lower incisors should be borne in mind.

It must be stressed that palatal and lingual arches as described will not guarantee against forward movement of molars. Cases in which they are used must be regularly inspected not only for appliance breakage but also for evidence of unwanted movement. The possibility of irritation caused by a palatal arch or of lower-incisor proclination caused by a lingual arch should be remembered.

Palatal and lingual arches may need to be in place for many months. The bands must of course be well fitting, and attention must be paid to routine band servicing.

## CONSTRUCTION

These arches are made in the laboratory on a model. The model is made from an impression which is taken with the bands seated on the molars. The bands are removed and replaced in the impression so that the working model carries the bands themselves in their correct position.

The arches are soldered to the bands to make a rigid appliance for space maintenance. Alternatively, where the arch will need to be activated, it may be made removable by attaching it to the lingual surfaces of the molars by a locking device. The locking devices which are most useful are the McKeag system and the Selmer–Olsen system (*Fig.* 7.3).

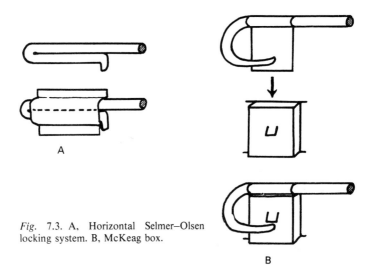

*Fig.* 7.3. A, Horizontal Selmer–Olsen locking system. B, McKeag box.

The arch itself is most commonly made in 0·8 or 0·9 mm diameter hard stainless-steel wire.

Palatal arches can be improved by the addition of an acrylic button incorporated in the anterior section. Although this cannot be removed for cleaning by the patient, it seldom causes appreciable irritation to the palate in practice. It should be kept well free of the margins of the teeth and not extended so that the lower incisors occlude with it (*Fig.* 7.4).

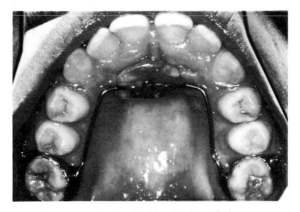

*Fig.* 7.4. Palatal arch with palatal acrylic button.

## Sectional Fixed Space Maintainers

The need occasionally arises to preserve space for a single unerupted tooth when it seems inappropriate to fit a lingual or palatal arch. In

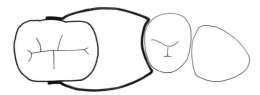

*Fig.* 7.5. Sectional space maintainer, soldered to a band on lower first molar.

such a case one of the teeth adjacent to the space is banded and a rigid arm is then soldered to the band. The arm spans the space without impeding eruption of the unerupted tooth (*Fig.* 7.5).

### REFERENCE

Friel S. and McKeag H. T. A. (1939) *Dent. Rec.* **59,** 359.

# CHAPTER 8

# EXTRA-ORAL TRACTION

In the treatment of many malocclusions intra-oral anchorage is insufficient to enable the required tooth movements to be achieved. To overcome this problem extra-oral forces are used to supplement the intra-oral anchorage.

The force is provided by elastics, or springs, attached to a headcap or neckstrap. The force is transmitted to the arches either by a bow which engages into tubes on molar bands, or by two separate wires which hook onto the anterior part of the archwire. The magnitude of the force can be varied by the degree of activation of the elastics or springs of the headcap. Much higher forces than can be derived solely from intra-oral anchorage are possible.

The direction in which the force is applied can be varied, and is mainly dependent upon the type of headcap, or neckstrap used. The direction of extra-oral force used should be chosen after consideration of the tooth movements required to achieve a satisfactory result.

The duration of wear of extra-oral force can be varied according to the needs of the occlusion, but a minimum amount of wear is for 12 hours out of every 24, with the normal amount of wear being 14 hours out of every 24 hours. Good patient co-operation is essential for adequate wear.

## *Method of Applying Extra-oral Force*

The force is generated by stretching the elastic or spring elements of a headcap. Elastic force can be provided either by the use of replaceable elastic bands, or by elasticated material. Various patterns and sizes of neckstrap and headcap are available commercially.

The direction of force that can be provided is described as high pull, straight pull (occipital), or low pull (cervical) (*Fig.* 8.1). High pull and straight pull can only be produced by a headcap; low pull is provided by a neckstrap. The cervical neckstrap has an advantage in that it is less conspicuous than a headcap, but it should only be used if the direction of pull that it provides is appropriate to the malocclusion under treatment.

The force is transmitted to the dental arches in one of two ways:

1. By means of an extra-oral arch, which fits into tubes welded onto molar bands.

2. By the use of two hooks which engage the anterior part of the archwire, and which are called 'J' hooks by virtue of their shape.

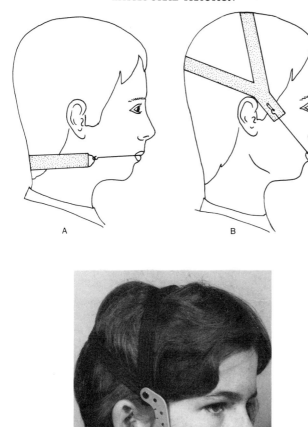

*Fig.* 8.1. A, Low-pull neckstrap. B, High-pull headcap. C, Variable pull headcap being used for straight pull.

## Extra-oral Arch

The extra-oral arch is made of two elements: an inner labial arch which engages in tubes on molar bands, and an outer extra-oral arch which hooks onto the neckstrap or headcap (*Fig.* 8.2) (Klöehn, 1947). Preformed extra-oral arches are available in a variety of sizes.

59

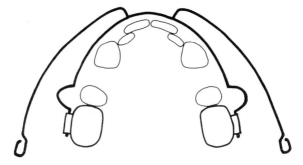

*Fig.* 8.2. An extra-oral arch with U-loops. The inner arch of 1·15 mm diameter fits into 1·15 mm internal diameter buccal tubes.

INNER ARCH: The authors find that the inner arch is best made of 1·15 mm hard stainless-steel wire. It slides into buccal tubes on upper molar bands. These tubes are positioned occlusally to the tubes taking the archwire, and parallel to them. Preformed double buccal tubes are available, which must be firmly welded to the band to prevent separation by the forces applied.

There are various ways in which the arch may be stopped at the mesial aspect of the buccal tube, so that the force is transmitted to the molars. Bayonet offsets or U-loops are commonly used for this purpose (*Fig.* 8.3). U-loops have the advantage that they allow for adjustment to increase the anteroposterior length of the inner arch during treatment. This is necessary when the upper molars are being moved distally, in order to clear the bow from the incisors.

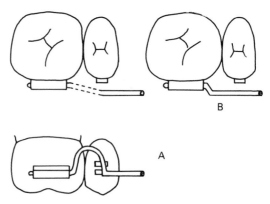

*Fig.* 8.3. Stops on inner arch of extra-oral appliance. A, U-loop. B, Horizontal bayonet bend.

OUTER ARCH: This is made in 1·5 mm diameter stainless-steel wire.

The arch is bent round parallel to the surface of the cheeks. Hooks for the attachment of the extra-oral force are bent opposite the first molars, approximately 3 cm in front of the lobes of the ears.

FITTING AN EXTRA-ORAL ARCH: The inner arch should be made initially so that it lies passively in the molar tubes. Stops or U-loops must be adjusted so that the bow does not touch the incisors or any of the buccal teeth apart from the molars. The junction of the inner and outer elements should lie between the lips when they are comfortably held together. The extra-oral arch should not press into the patient's face, and must be free of sharp edges.

The patient must demonstrate that he can insert the appliance correctly.

The force applied should be about 500 g initially, and the patient is warned to expect some discomfort. The patient must be encouraged to wear the appliance as much as possible—it should be worn for not less than 12 hours per day.

## J Hooks

The extra-oral force is transmitted from the headcap by a separate wire on each side. The wires terminate anteriorly in hooks which engage the labial span of the archwire directly (*Fig.* 8.4). The wire hooks are constructed so that they pass forwards away from the archwire, out of the mouth, and terminate in hooks that rest on the cheek at about the first molar region. The posterior ends of the J

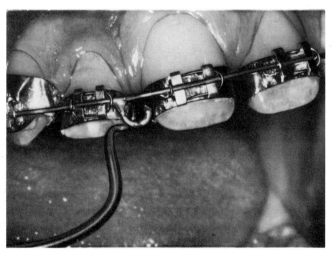

*Fig.* 8.4. Extra-oral force applied directly to the archwire.

hooks are supported by the headcap, and elastics are stretched between the headcap and J hook.

### Direction of Force

Although the principal use of extra-oral force is to reinforce intra-oral anchorage, it is possible during treatment involving extra-oral anchorage to influence anterior facial height, and the vertical position

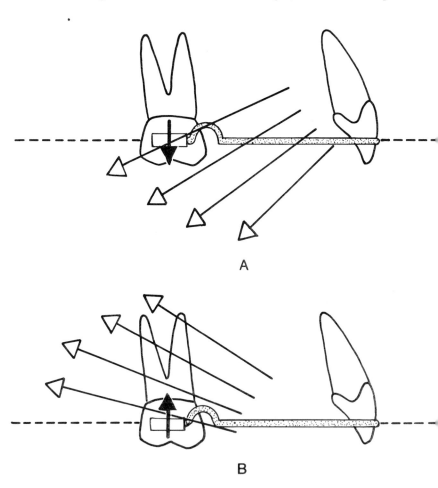

A

B

*Fig.* 8.5. The effect of direction of extra-oral force when used for distal movement of molars: A, Force direction leading to extrusion of molars with secondary 'clockwise' rotation of the mandible. B, Force direction leading to intrusion of molars.

of the upper labial segment. The effect of extra-oral force on the facial skeleton is related to the direction of the applied force.

The anterior facial height is influenced by the vertical height of the molars. Extrusion of the upper molars increases the maxillary mandibular planes angle and thus causes the mandible to be slightly more retruded. When an extra-oral bow is used, and the direction of the force points backwards and downwards relative to the occlusal plane, extrusion of molars occurs. Extrusion of molars commonly occurs when a cervical neckstrap is used with an extra-oral bow (*Fig.* 8.5A).

The movement of the mandible that results from the extrusion of molars is called 'clockwise rotation'. (This description assumes that the patient is viewed from the right-hand side.)

Intrusion of molars during the use of extra-oral forces can only be achieved when a headcap is used in conjunction with an extra-oral arch. The direction of force must be backwards and upwards relative to the occlusal plane (*Fig.* 8.5B).

Intrusion of upper incisors can be achieved using J hooks attached directly to the anterior part of the maxillary archwire, and with the extra-oral force applied upwards and backwards with a high-pull headgear.


# USES OF EXTRA-ORAL ANCHORAGE

The principal use of extra-oral force is to provide additional anchorage, when the anchorage that can be derived solely from intra-oral forces is insufficient to carry out the required tooth movements. Extra-oral anchorage can also be used to carry out certain specific tooth movements.

The possible uses of extra-oral anchorage are:
1. Anchorage reinforcement.
2. Distal movement of upper molars.
3. Space maintenance.
4. Canine retraction.
5. Overjet reduction.

*Anchorage Reinforcement*
When anchorage reinforcement is required extra-oral forces can be applied to the upper arch by means of an extra-oral arch, or to either the upper or lower arch using J hooks.

With an extra-oral arch the aim of anchorage reinforcement is to prevent forward movement of the molars to which the extra-oral arch is attached. Canine retraction and overjet reduction can then be carried out without forward movement of the upper buccal segments.

When using J hooks for anchorage reinforcement the extra-oral force is transmitted directly to the archwire. Tooth movements within the arch are carried out using intramaxillary forces.

Intermaxillary elastic traction may be used in conjunction with extra-oral forces with either Class II, or Class III traction. Class III traction can be used to 'transmit' extra-oral force to the lower arch, as an alternative to applying extra-oral force directly to the lower arch.

### Distal Movement of Upper Molars

Space may be provided for alignment of anterior teeth by distal movement of upper first molars. This is often combined with the extraction of upper second molars, which makes the distal movement of first molars easier. It is best carried out before correction of the labial segment is commenced, so that all the extra-oral force is utilized in the distal movement and not dissipated in providing anchorage for tooth movements further forward in the arch.

MANAGEMENT OF DISTAL MOVEMENT:

1. Where distal movement of molars is required both the force applied and the amount of wear are important. The total force should be approximately 1500 g.

2. Extra-oral traction should never be worn for less than 12 hours in any day. The longer the patient can wear it the better. Most patients of school age can be expected to be at home for 14 hours a day and this time is therefore a useful target to ask the patient to achieve.

3. As the molars move distally they must also move buccally to be accommodated in the greater width of the dental arch (*Fig.* 8.6). Failure to do this may produce a bilateral cross-bite on the molars. Intermolar width expansion is produced by activating the inner bow of

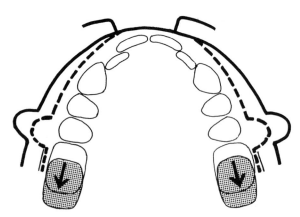

*Fig.* 8.6. When 6|6 move distally they must also move buccally. The inner arch of the extra-oral appliance is expanded to achieve this.

the extra-oral arch. The amount of expansion on the inner bow is checked by inserting first one side and then the other; the side not engaged should rest 3–5 mm buccally to the molar tube. This method of expansion may also be used to correct an established molar crossbite.

4. As the molars move distally the bow will impinge against the incisors, so that it becomes necessary to lengthen the inner arch. With U-adjustment loops this is a simple matter. If bayonet bends have been used to 'stop' the arch in front of the molar tubes, only a small amount of adjustment is possible, and it may be necessary to solder stops on to the archwire in order to prevent it sliding too far into the molar tubes.

5. Check the occlusion and ensure that distal movement is not being hampered by interference from the lower molars. If this happens a removable appliance with an anterior bite plane can help.

UNILATERAL DISTAL MOVEMENT: By adjustment of the outer arm of the extra-oral arch it is possible to alter the relative force on the molars. Both the point at which the elastic traction is applied and the angle at which the force is delivered to the extra-oral arch influence the distribution of the applied load to the molars.

In practice there are two ways of increasing the distal force on a particular molar:

1. Increase the length of the arm on the side where most distal movement is required.

2. Increase the angle between the outer bow and the side of the face, so that before the traction is applied the hook stands away from the cheek on the side that most movement is required (*Fig. 8.7*).

MOLAR TIPPING: When upper molars are being moved distally by means of an extra-oral arch, the teeth either tip distally, or bodily movement occurs. The response of a tooth depends upon the direction in which the force is applied. The direction of force may be controlled by choice of an appropriate headcap, by adjustment of the angle of the outer arch relative to the inner arch, or by altering the length of the outer arm (*Fig. 8.8*).

In general, (provided that the extra-oral arm is longer than the inner arch) if the outer arm is angled upwards, relative to the inner arch, distal movement of the apices is encouraged. If distal movement of the crown is to be encouraged the outer arm should be angled downwards relative to the inner arch. In theory it should be possible to achieve bodily distal movement of the molars, but this is difficult to achieve in practice.

MOLAR ROTATION: When upper molars move forward spontaneously they usually rotate around their palatal root. By activation of the inner bow of an extra-oral arch it is possible to 'derotate' a molar. Careful adjustment of the distal end of the inner arch is made so that it lies at a

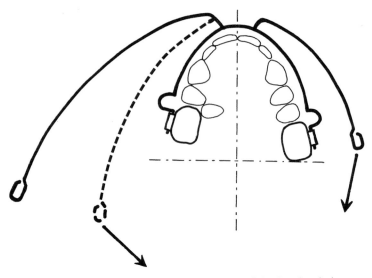

*Fig.* 8.7. To apply a greater force on one side of the dental arch the outer arm of the extra-oral appliance is made longer and bent away from the cheek. When the neckstrap is engaged the longer arm is brought close to the cheek, and a greater force is applied to the tooth on that side.

slight angle to the molar tube. This is checked by inserting the inner arch only into the tube on the molar to be rotated. The stop on the opposite side should lie just distally to the molar tube on that side. When the arch is inserted into both molar tubes a rotational force is then applied (*Fig.* 8.9).

### Space Maintenance
Extra-oral traction may be used to prevent forward movement of upper molars following the extraction of permanent teeth. It is used in preference to, or in addition to, a palatal arch when additional anchorage will be required for tooth movement at a later stage.

### Canine Retraction
Either maxillary or mandibular canines can be retracted using J hooks; these are placed over the archwire and the hook contacts the mesial aspect of the canine bracket (p. 80). The canines are thus moved distally along the archwire.

### Incisor Retraction
J HOOKS: These can be used in conjunction with an archwire with closing loops to reduce an overjet. At the same time some incisor in-

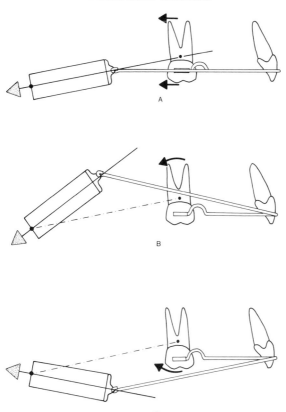

*Fig.* 8.8. Molar tipping during distal movement of 6|6 with an extra-oral arch. A, If the direction on the applied force passes through the centre of resistance of 6|6, bodily movement occurs. B, If the direction of the applied force passes above the centre of resistance of 6|6, distal apex tipping occurs. C, If the direction of the applied force passes below the centre of resistance of 6|6, distal crown tipping occurs.

trusion can be achieved if high pull forces are used.

**EXTRA-ORAL ARCH:** When an extra-oral arch is being used to move upper molars distally, a degree of spontaneous improvement in the crowding of anterior teeth is often seen. Where there is an increased overjet some reduction of this may occur as the buccal segments move distally.

Overjet reduction can be carried out solely with extra-oral traction when the overbite is incomplete. A latex elastic is stretched across hooks on the inner arch of the bow (*Fig.* 8.10). The elastic rests

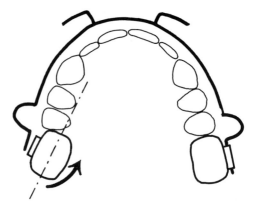

*Fig.* 8.9. Extra-oral arch to produce derotation of an upper molar. The angle between the molar tube and the inner arch should be small to ensure that the patient can insert the appliance.

against the labial surfaces of the incisors. An advantage of this system is that the anchorage of the upper buccal segments is not used for the reduction of overjet. When the upper incisors are very proclined, however, it is difficult to prevent the elastic from sliding upwards into contact with the gingivae. Since the elastic is stretched between two points it is impossible to control accurately the labiolingual position of the upper incisors. In addition, considerable distal tipping of incisors, associated with labial movement of their apices, may be seen when an elastic is used in this way to reduce an overjet.

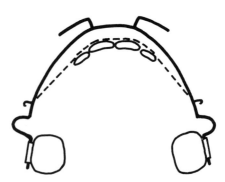

*Fig.* 8.10. Extra-oral appliance with an anterior elastic for reduction of an overjet.

## *Extra-oral Anchorage to the Mandibular Arch*

This is normally best applied by means of J hooks. If extra-oral anchorage is already in use in the upper arch, anchorage reinforcement can be provided by using Class III intermaxillary traction at the same time (*Fig.* 8.11). Class III traction is normally applied by elastics running between hooks on the upper molar bands and archwire hooks lying hard against the mesial surfaces of the lower canine brackets. If the lower molars require distal movement, sliding jigs can be used to transmit the intermaxillary traction directly to the lower molars. When Class III traction is used in this way the amount of anchorage provided by the extra-oral traction for use in the upper arch is, of course, reduced; and if space in the upper arch is critical it is necessary to apply the Class III traction only when the extra-oral traction apparatus is being worn.

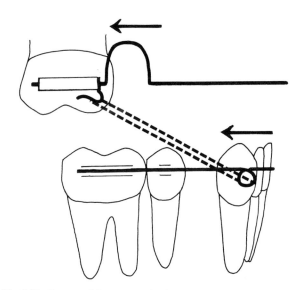

*Fig.* 8.11. Extra-oral force transmitted to the lower archwire by means of Class III elastic traction.

## PATIENT SUPERVISION

It must be emphasized that the effectiveness of extra-oral traction is largely dependent upon the patient's co-operation. Resistance on the part of the patient to wearing the apparatus is easy to understand as it is both inconvenient and unsightly, and frequently causes some discomfort in the teeth to which it is applied.

The most important point is to persuade the patient to wear the extra-oral traction for a sufficient period each day. For this reason it is helpful to present it as an appliance that need not be worn at school or work, but which should be worn for the rest of the time, when at home, including when asleep. Some patients are prepared to wear extra-oral traction full time.

When distal movement of upper molars is required the patient should be encouraged to wear extra-oral traction as much as possible. He can be asked to keep a record of the hours that the appliance is worn each day.

If only a limited amount of extra-oral traction is required its wear can be restricted to the sleeping hours. It is extremely difficult, however, to get a patient to increase the amount of wear once a regular pattern has been established.

If extra-oral traction is going to be required during treatment it is advisable to use it from the beginning of active treatment.

*Assessment of Wear*

Since extra-oral traction depends so heavily upon patient co-operation, it is vitally important at each visit to be able to assess whether the apparatus has been worn sufficiently. If the patient realizes that the orthodontist is not aware of whether the appliance is worn or not, co-operation is unlikely to be very satisfactory.

QUESTIONS TO PATIENT: Each operator will have methods of assessing removable-appliance wear, and similar principles apply with questions about wear of extra-oral traction. Leading questions such as, 'Are you wearing it for 14 hours every day?' invite the reply 'Yes'. It is better to make the patient defend his position—for example, determine when the patient goes to bed and gets up and then say. 'That only makes 10 hours wear', to which the patient will either look uncomfortable or reply, 'The appliance is inserted some hours before going to bed'.

OBSERVATION OF PATIENT AND APPLIANCE: Ask the patient to insert the appliance; those who are wearing it regularly will have little difficulty in doing this, probably without using a mirror. Good co-operation can be checked by inspecting the headcap or neckstrap, which should give the appearance of having been worn. It may have taken on a curved form and have lost some of its elasticity. In view of the fact that relapse of molar position may occur if the extra-oral traction is not worn, the patient must be instructed to contact the orthodontist as soon as possible should the appliance be lost or broken.

OBSERVATION OF THE OCCLUSION: In addition to the patient's conscious reaction to the appliance, the following pointers to adequate wear are of use:

1. Mobility. Molars to which extra-oral forces are applied should become slightly mobile.

2. Tooth movement. In the early stages, the initial reference models are used to refer back to in assessing molar movement; later, direct measurements are useful. Dividers can be used to record the distance between the mesial ends of the molar tubes and, for instance, the mesio-incisal angles of the upper incisors. This does not provide a very accurate measurement, but it is better than no measurement at all. If the upper incisors are used as a reference point, it should be borne in mind that they may move during treatment. Sometimes the overjet will be seen to reduce spontaneously when extra-oral traction is applied to upper molars, even if no force is applied to the incisors by the appliance.

## REFERENCES

Armstrong M. M. (1971) *Am. J. Orthod.* **59,** 217.
Berman M. (1976) *Br. J. Orthod.* **3,** 131.
Gianelly A. (1971) *Am. J. Orthod.* **60,** 257.
Haack D. C. (1963) *Am. J. Orthod.* **49,** 330.
Klöehn J. (1947) *Angle Orthod.* **17,** 10.
Oosthuizen L., Dijkman J. P. F. and Evans W. G., *Angle Orthod.* **43,** 221.
Sandusky W. C. (1965) *Am. J. Orthod.* **51,** 262.

CHAPTER 9

# CANINE ALIGNMENT

Most orthodontic patients seek treatment to improve the appearance of their anterior teeth. The alignment of incisors and canines is thus a most important part of orthodontic treatment.

For the purposes of description, canine alignment and incisor alignment will be described in separate chapters, although in practice both movements are often achieved simultaneously.

The alignment of canines is not concerned merely with the correction of their axial inclination and their lateral, rotational, and vertical position. The relationship of upper and lower canines in occlusion is important, as is the position of the canines relative to the incisors. A common problem with maxillary canines is failure of eruption due to palatal or buccal displacement. Such teeth often require a fixed appliance to bring them into correct alignment.

## DISTAL MOVEMENT OF CANINES

In cases in which there is crowding of the incisors, the canines will usually be in a position which prevents alignment of the incisors within the space available. If an increased overjet is to be reduced by palatal movement of the upper incisor crowns, this movement is in most cases not possible without causing crowding of the incisors unless the canines are moved distally.

In the upper arch distal movement of canines is therefore usually necessary both for relief of incisor crowding and also to make space for overjet reduction. Canines have long roots and a relatively large root area, and great care must therefore be taken during canine retraction to avoid unwanted movement of the anchor teeth (*see* Chapter 13).

The position of the canines in the lower arch is an important guide to the final stable position of an occlusion under treatment. With the lower labial segment in a stable uncrowded position it is usually necessary to retract the upper canines into a Class I relationship, in order to obtain enough space to align the upper incisors and reduce the overjet. Space for alignment of the canines must not be created by overexpansion of intercanine width, which is liable to relapse. The inclination of the canine relative to the occlusal plane is important when considering distal movement of a canine.

## Mesially Inclined Canines

If a distally directed force is applied to the crown of a mesially inclined canine, and the tooth is free to tip, it will become less mesially inclined as the crown moves distally away from the incisors. When a canine is slightly mesially inclined and the amount of distal movement of the crown that is required is not great, retraction by means of a distally directed tipping force may result in a satisfactory alignment of the canine. If, however, the amount of distal crown movement required is considerable, the canine may be severely distally inclined at the completion of canine retraction, and uprighting will be required.

Spontaneous distal movement of mesially inclined canines occurs following first premolar extraction, particularly in the lower arch. In mildly crowded cases this may allow an appreciable amount of spontaneous lower incisor alignment.

## Upright Canines

A canine which is neither mesially nor distally inclined requires as much distal movement of the apex as of the crown. This is achieved either by distal tipping, followed by uprighting, or by bodily retraction. In either case, more anchorage is required than for distal tipping alone.

## Distally Inclined Canines

Distally inclined canines must be retracted with more distal movement of the apex than of the crown. Such movement requires a considerable amount of anchorage (*Fig. 9.1*). The tooth must first be uprighted by distal movement of the apex and then retracted bodily.

The following methods are available for canine retraction:

## Upper Removable Appliances

Removable appliances produce tooth movement principally by tipping. Upper removable appliances are therefore useful for retracting mesially inclined upper canines. They may be used in the early stages of the treatment of cases which will eventually require a fully banded appliance. If extra-oral traction is required it can be applied to bands on the first permanent molars, the removable appliance being fitted with retention clasps which engage the undercuts above the molar tubes (*Fig. 9.2*).

Upper removable appliances find their main use for retracting canines when the upper incisors are well aligned but an increased overjet is present. When the upper incisors are severely rotated, they are banded early in treatment and the canines are retracted using a fixed appliance mechanism.

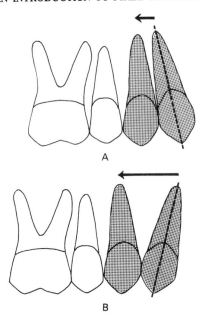

*Fig.* 9.1. A, Retraction of mesially inclined canine. B, Retraction of a distally inclined canine, showing the amount of distal movement of the apex which is required.

## Sectional Archwires

Canine retraction can be achieved by using a short sectional archwire which extends forwards from the molar tube to the canine. The incisors are not banded. The retracting force is applied to the canine by intramaxillary traction, and the canine moves *with* the archwire, rather than *along* it.

### Indications

1. Canines which are upright or distally inclined before retraction need to be retracted with the apex moving further distally than the crown. This movement consumes a considerable amount of anchorage, and it may be necessary to concentrate the available anchorage in the correction of the canine position rather than retracting the canine and, for example, reducing the overjet at the same time. A sectional archwire may therefore be used to retract and align such canines. The archwire may be activated to produce apical movement and rotation at the same time as distal movement.

2. Occasionally cases are seen in which canine retraction alone is all that is required to complete treatment. There may be sufficient

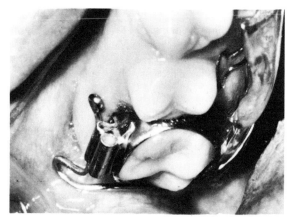

*Fig.* 9.2. Clasp on removable appliance for fitting over 6|6 bands.

spontaneous improvement in incisor position to avoid the necessity for these teeth to be banded. In such cases sectional archwires may be used as an alternative to banding every tooth in the arch.

*Construction*

Rectangular wire is the most suitable material for the construction of sectional archwires designed to retract canines (*see Fig.* 9.3). The advantages of using rectangular wire are:

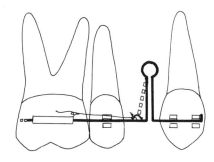

*Fig.* 9.3. Rectangular sectional archwire for canine retraction, showing activation by a tie-back ligature.

1. The relative rigidity of the rectangular wire means that the buccopalatal position of the canine can be controlled and sufficient force applied to produce apical movement if required.

2. Because the rectangular wire fits into rectangular bracket channels, the archwire cannot rotate in the brackets.

Edgewise brackets and attachments must be placed on the molar, second premolar, and canine.

75

It is advisable to place lingual buttons or cleats on the canine and molar bands so that lingual or palatal elastic traction can be applied during distal movement. This helps to reduce the possibility of rotation of the canine which may occur when using sectional canine retractors.

Initially, a roundwire sectional may be required in order to obtain full bracket engagement of the second premolar. Failure to incorporate the second premolar in the sectional may result in excessive forward movement of the first molar during canine retraction.

To retract a canine with a sectional archwire intramaxillary traction is applied by means of a closing loop (*Fig.* 9.4). There are a number of

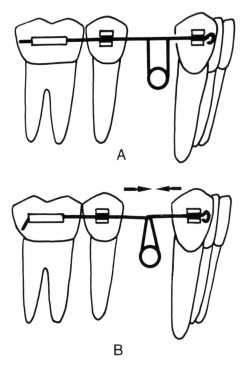

*Fig.* 9.4. Activation of a canine retraction sectional. A, Passive. B, Active.

different designs of closing loop, and to increase their flexibility the thickness of the loop may be reduced by selective electrolytic reduction.

The closing loop should be constructed close to the canine so that it can be reactivated progressively as the canine is retracted. A soldered hook may be placed just distal to the closing loop to enable activation by means of a tie-back ligature. In order to reduce the amount of tip-

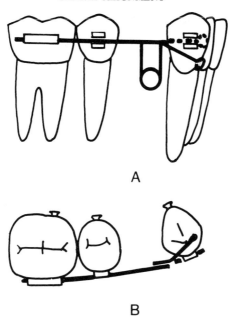

A

B

*Fig.* 9.5. Canine retraction sectional. A, Anti-tip bend. B, Anti-rotation bend.

ping or rotation of the canine, anti-tip and anti-rotation bends are incorporated in the mesial arm of the sectional (*Fig.* 9.5).

If a canine is distally inclined it should be uprighted prior to retraction by progressive adjustment of the mesial arm of the sectional. The reaction to the distal movement of the canine apex is mesial movement of the crown, which should be prevented by slight activation of the closing loop. When the canine is upright, an anti-tip bend is made in the sectional, and canine retraction is begun.

Canine retraction requires a considerable amount of anchorage and extra-oral anchorage will usually be necessary, especially when the canine is distally inclined before retraction. When using canine retraction sectionals the extra-oral anchorage must be provided by means of a facebow to double buccal tubes on the molars.

*Limitations of Sectional Arches*

Cases in which the correction of canine position alone is sufficient to complete treatment are relatively rare. In most cases, therefore, if bands are to be used at all, the whole arch can be banded and greater control over tooth position thereby obtained.

77

When a sectional arch is used the canine is at the end of a relatively long 'arm', and the control of the tooth's movement comes from its distal aspect only. When a 'full' archwire is used movement is controlled from both mesial and distal aspects, and there is therefore more control of rotational, apical, and buccopalatal movement.

To avoid unwanted tooth movements great care must be exercised in adjusting sectional archwires.

### *Canine Retraction along the Archwire*

Canines can be moved distally along a 'base' archwire by the application of a distally directed force to the canine. When the canine moves it does so by tipping. As a result of this tipping the archwire channel of an edgewise bracket lies at an angle to the archwire, and binding occurs between the archwire and the bracket. Part of the force used to retract the canine will thus be dissipated in overcoming this friction. If the forces used for canine retraction have been derived intra-orally, bracket binding can easily lead to an undesirable loss of space.

In order to keep bracket binding to a minimum, an archwire which engages the bracket closely without being a tight fit should be used (*Fig.* 9.6). Canine retraction along the archwire should therefore not be commenced until a base archwire of 0·4 mm can be fitted. Smaller diameter archwires or multistrand archwires should not be used when retracting canines because they allow excessive tipping and bracket binding to occur.

There are a number of ways to produce the retracting force:

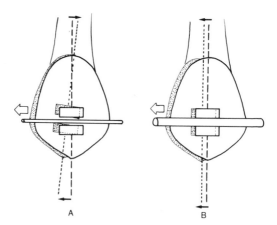

*Fig.* 9.6. Canine retraction along an archwire. A, If a narrower diameter archwire is used the canine tips, and binding occurs. B, Bracket binding is minimized if the archwire is a closer fit in the bracket.

## Elastics

Elastic traction can be applied directly to the bracket on the canine. If elastic ligature is used the canine should be tied loosely to the archwire with a stainless-steel ligature. The elastic ligature is passed in front of the bracket and tied back to the first molar. If a linked bracket elastic is used the loops should be placed over the canine and second premolar bracket and hooked onto the buccal hook on the first molar. However, both bracket elastics and elastic ligature increase the frictional forces between the canine bracket and the archwire. Linked bracket elastics or elastic thread can be used simultaneously on the lingual or palatal aspect to aid in canine retraction.

Latex elastic loops can be used to retract canines, but in order to achieve this a preformed ligature with an extension which forms a hook for the attachment of the elastic must be used on the canine. Anteriorly the elastic is hooked over the canine ligature instead of an archwire hook. Either Class II or Class III intermaxillary traction can be used in this manner.

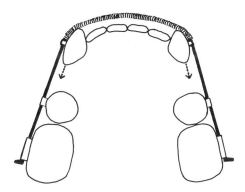

*Fig.* 9.7. Archwire, 0·45 mm, with compressed coil spring to retract $\overline{3|3}$. $\overline{21|12}$ are not banded. The archwire must be turned down distal to 6|6.

## Coil Springs

Compressed coil springs can be used to retract canines. *Fig.* 9.7 shows an appliance in which the incisors are not banded and a long coil spring is compressed between the canines. The distal ends of the archwire are turned down as they emerge from the molar tubes to prevent the archwire from being displaced forwards. The molars thus provide the anchorage against which the canines are moved distally. The canines must slide distally along the archwire. If edgewise brackets are used binding is likely to occur, but this is reduced if the archwire is a close fit in the bracket.

79

If Begg brackets are used, the canines will tip distally along the archwire. There is a danger that the intercanine width will be excessively increased when a coil spring is used in this way, unless the archwire is actively 'contracted' in the canine areas.

### Extra-oral Force

Extra-oral traction is an efficient method of retracting canines along an archwire. As the forces for canine movement are derived extraorally, any bracket binding transmits a distally directed force to the archwire and there is no forward movement of the posterior teeth as a reaction to the canine retraction. In order to apply the extra-oral force directly to the canines, it is necessary to use J hooks (Chapter 8) which are hooked over the archwire and engage the mesial aspect of the canine brackets (*Fig.* 9.8). A straight-pull headgear provides the

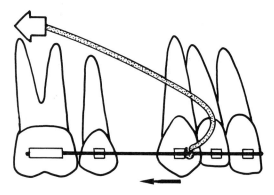

*Fig.* 9.8.   Canine retraction with extra-oral force. J hooks are engaged over the archwire, in contact with the mesial bracket on the canine.

optimum direction of force. It is possible to retract all four canines sumultaneously using this method, with a pair of J hooks on each side of the mouth.

### Canine Retraction with Active Archwires

Distal movement of canines can be carried out with looped archwires. In this case the canine moves with the archwire, and there is therefore no problem with bracket binding (*Fig.* 9.9).

When the labial segment is well aligned a vertical loop may be placed on either side of the canine with the distal limb of the anterior loop in contact with the mesial of the canine bracket. In the labial section the archwire lies just forwards of the incisor brackets. The

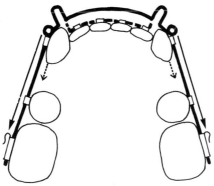

*Fig.* 9.9. Archwire, 0·40 mm, to retract 3|3. The labial section is tied into 21|12 and intramaxillary elastics are applied between the archwire hooks and 6|6.

archwire is activated by tying it into the brackets on the incisors and by pulling the archwire through the molar tubes (*Fig.* 9.10). Where the incisors are crowded, multilooped archwires can be used to produce canine retraction and incisor alignment simultaneously. Anchorage reinforcement is often required to prevent undue proclination of incisors during this movement. When Begg brackets are used canine retraction, incisor alignment, and overjet reduction can be carried out simultaneously, utilizing intermaxillary traction. The free tipping that can take place with Begg brackets enables these movements to take place relatively rapidly. However, the canines may require uprighting after they have been tipped distally.

The use of mutilooped archwires to produce canine retraction and incisor alignment sumultaneously is described fully on p. 93.

## ROTATION OF CANINES

The rotational position of a canine can be changed either by using an active section of the archwire or by using elastics.

When the archwire is used to produce rotation of a canine it is preferable to use a bracket of appreciable mesiodistal width, the section of the archwire lying in the bracket being adjusted to apply a rotational moment to the tooth. Alternatively, elastic ligature attached to a lingual button can be used to rotate canines.

Canines often require rotation as well as distal movement. When the canine is severely rotated, its rotational position will need to be corrected prior to distal movement. With less severe rotations the archwire mechanisms which have been described for distal movement of canines can also be adjusted to correct the rotation during distal movement.

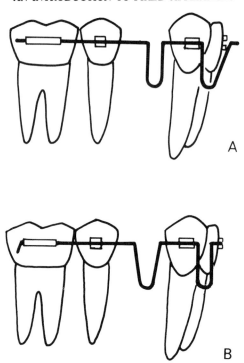

*Fig*. 9.10. An archwire to retract 3|3. A, Passive. B, Active.

## BUCCOLINGUAL MOVEMENT OF CANINES

Control of intercanine width is very important. If canines are to be moved distally on to a wider part of the arch, they may also need to be moved laterally. Overexpansion of intercanine width, however, is likely to relapse. A common finding in crowded arches is that the canines are displaced too far buccally. In these cases the intercanine width may need to be maintained, or even reduced, during canine retraction.

The movement of canines in a lingual direction can be difficult, particularly in the lower arch, where the relatively small incisor roots provide little anchorage. *Fig*. 9.11 illustrates an archwire activated to move both lower canines in a lingual direction. In this case the canines provide reciprocal anchorage.

To ensure that an archwire will not produce expansion of intercanine width it should be placed in the molar tubes and then checked to make sure that it lies in the canine brackets rather than standing away from them.

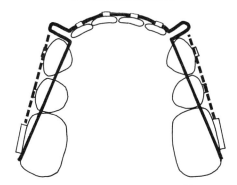

*Fig.* 9.11. Archwire, 0·40 mm, to move 3|3 lingually.

The retraction of upper canines which are in Class II relationship is sometimes prevented by the position of the lower canines. When the teeth are in occlusion the lower canine or its bracket occludes with the upper canine in such a way as to prevent distal movement. This problem can be overcome by temporarily moving the upper canine buccally or the lower canine lingually, and then completing canine alignment.

## UPRIGHTING OF PREMOLARS AND CANINES

The space provided by the extraction of first premolars is utilized in the following ways:

1. By distal movement of canines, which will provide space for alignment of incisors.

2. By mesial movement of the teeth distal to the site of extraction.

The proportion of the extraction space used in each of these ways during treatment must be carefully controlled. The amount of mesial movement of teeth distal to the extraction space must not be so great as to prevent alignment of the anterior teeth.

The occlusion of the buccal teeth is important not only from the point of view of caries susceptibility and periodontal considerations, but also from the point of view of the stability of the orthodontic result.

If during orthodontic treatment the extraction space has been closed, with the second premolars mesially inclined, the space will tend to re-establish itself as the canines and premolars upright spontaneously following removal of the appliance. The canine uprighting may then result in deterioration in the position of the incisors.

If reopening of the extraction space is to be prevented, it is important that the roots of canines and second premolars are parallel, or even convergent apically, at the completion of treatment.

The amount of tipping of canines and premolars that occurs during canine retraction and closure of premolar extraction space depends upon the mechanism used.

With edgewise brackets, if bodily canine retraction is carried out either with sectional archwires or by retraction along the archwire, the amount of uprighting required is minimal. Uprighting can be achieved by the use of progressively more rigid archwires, incorporating bends to move the apices together.

If a looped archwire is used to retract canines and close extraction spaces a certain amount of tipping can occur as a result of flexibility of the archwire. The archwire should be adjusted on either side of the extraction space so that distal movement of the canine apex and mesial movement of the second premolar apex is encouraged. In some instances when the extraction space has been closed it may be necessary to revert to a smaller diameter plain archwire and achieve uprighting by progressive increase in archwire dimension. It is vital to tie the canine and premolar together during this stage to ensure that the extraction space does not reopen during the uprighting.

## Begg Uprighting Springs

When Begg brackets are used a considerable amount of tipping occurs. Uprighting is then achieved with uprighting springs which are very effective and once in position do not usually require reactivation. They are available preformed, and incorporate a helical coil. One arm is passed through the vertical channel of the Begg bracket and the other engages the archwire.

The movements which may be produced by these uprighting springs are:

1. Crown movements rather than apical movement (*Fig.* 9.12).

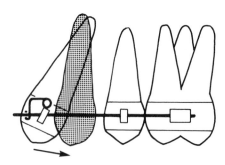

*Fig.* 9.12. An uprighting spring may be used to produce distal movement and improvement of axial inclination.

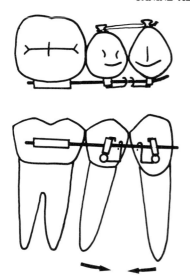

*Fig.* 9.13. Begg uprighting springs. Note that the crowns of 53⌐ are tied together and both teeth ligated to the archwire.

This movement can be prevented by tying the tooth to other teeth which have enough anchorage to resist movement. Where a tipped canine and premolar are in contact, reciprocal anchorage is utilized as their roots are paralleled, the crowns being tied together (*Fig.* 9.13).

2. Occlusal movement. The spring delivers an extruding force to the tooth. This must be prevented by tying the tooth onto the archwire.

The free end of the spring must be free to move along the archwire as the uprighting proceeds (*Fig.* 9.14). Care must be taken to ensure that uprighting springs do not inadvertently apply rotational forces.

## SEVERELY MISPLACED UPPER CANINES

The problems associated with the alignment of severely misplaced upper canines will be discussed on the assumption that the canine displacement is not such as to make alignment in the arch impossible or impracticable. It will also be assumed that there is enough space available for alignment, and that sufficient anchorage is available for the movement required.

### Palatally Misplaced Upper Canines
The buccal movement of palatally misplaced canines can be achieved either by 'pushing' the tooth from the palatal aspect (*Fig.* 9.15) or by

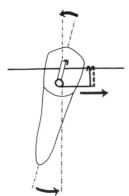

*Fig.* 9.14. As a tooth uprights the uprighting spring must be free to slide along the archwire.

'pulling' the tooth from the buccal aspect. In either case it will generally be necessary to provide a point of application for the force by cementing a band, or by using a direct-bonded attachment on the misplaced tooth. When a palatal spring is used the attachment offers a site for application of the spring. When buccal traction is being used the attachment provides a means of applying force to the tooth. It is generally preferable to move a palatally misplaced canine buccally by applying traction from the buccal aspect.

If the misplaced canine is only partially erupted it is often easier to use the other canine in the arch as a pattern for making the band. As an alternative to a band, a piece of contoured tape carrying a hook can be bonded directly to the tooth. It is sometimes not possible to attach a bracket to the band on a misplaced canine during the early stages of alignment. A hook or cleat can be used instead. Methods of applying traction to severely misplaced canines by means of 'pin' or 'lasso' have also been described.

When the canine is considerably displaced towards the midline, elastic ligature is tied between the canine and a buccal loop. If the canine needs to be rotated as well as moved buccally the attachment on the band is positioned accordingly. The elastic ligature must be replaced monthly (sooner if it breaks). The greater part of the buccal movement can be achieved by the use of elastic ligature. The archwire to which the elastic is attached must be of sufficient diameter to resist distortion (0·45 or 0·5 mm), and as many teeth as possible should be banded and attached to the archwire so as to provide sufficient anchorage.

As an alternative to elastic ligature, a flexible arm can be attached to the buccal surface of the molar band on the side where the misplaced canine lies, and ligature wire tied from the canine to the flexible arm so that a buccally directed force is applied to the canine. In this case there is a danger that the molar will be rotated mesiopalatally. Anchorage can be improved by the use of a palatal arch and extra-oral traction if necessary (*Fig. 9.15*).

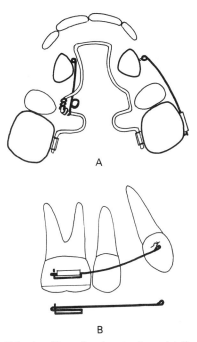

A

B

*Fig.* 9.15. A, Palatal and buccal springs to align palatally placed 3|3. B, Self-retaining buccal spring engaging buccal tube on molar band.

When the canine has been moved to within a short distance of its final buccopalatal position greater control of its position is achieved by attaching it to a buccal archwire. Sufficient flexibility in the length of archwire spanning the space into which the canine is to be moved is provided by vertical loops, small diameter archwire, or multistrand wire. The relatively rigid buccal archwire may be retained and the flexibility of fine or multistrand wire utilized by the addition of a small accessory archwire (*Fig.* 9.16), because of its flexibility in all planes. Final correction of the lateral and rotational position of the canine is achieved by the use of a looped section.

Sometimes a palatal canine is prevented from being moved buccally because of its occlusion with lower teeth. A lower removable

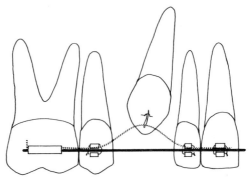

*Fig.* 9.16.  An accessory multistrand archwire to move 3| occlusally.

appliance incorporating posterior bite planes is useful for the short period during which the upper canine is moved 'over the bite'.

### Buccally Misplaced Canines

The alignment of buccally displaced canines usually involves retraction and occlusal movement, and sometimes rotation. When such canines lie over the upper laterals, they must be moved distally before being moved occlusally so that they are not brought into contact with the roots of the upper laterals (*Fig.* 9.17).

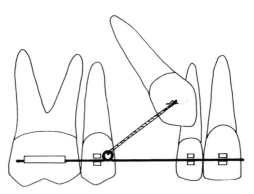

*Fig.* 9.17.  Elastic ligature used to move 3| distally and occlusally.

Disto-occlusal movement can be achieved by the attachment of elastic ligature to an archwire of sufficient diameter to resist distortion. When the canine has been moved far enough distally and is within a short distance of the archwire, an accessory arch made of fine wire or

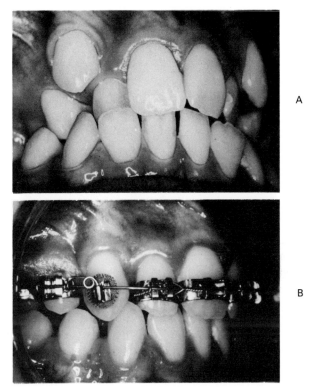

*Fig.* 9.18. A buccally placed canine. A, Before alignment. B, The canine has had a Begg bracket bonded onto it and an uprighting spring has been used to move the apex distally.

multistrand wire can then be used to move the tooth occlusally. Finally, the tooth can be attached to the main archwire for the completion of alignment (*Fig.* 9.18).

The occlusal movement of upper canines is very satisfactorily achieved by the use of an upper removable appliance (*Fig.* 9.19). The advantage of this method is that anchorage for the occlusal movement is provided by the large area of the palate in contact with the removable appliance, and unwanted tipping of teeth is minimized. A band carrying a hook is cemented to the canine, and the patient is instructed in the application of the flexible arm.

## Missing Upper Canines

When an upper canine is absent, it may be decided to move the upper buccal segment forward so that the upper first premolar can simulate

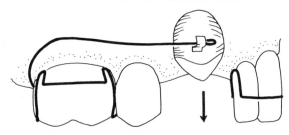

*Fig.* 9.19. A buccal spring on a removable appliance to move 3⌋ occlusally.

the missing canine. The premolars and molar are moved forward individually to close the available space completely. Coil springs or elastics may be used for moving the premolars forwards, and a closing loop on the archwire for the molar. Class III traction can be helpful for this mesial movement.

Every effort should be made (1) to close spaces completely and (2) to correct any mesial inclination which results from the forward movement of the buccal segment. If these points are not attended to, there is a likelihood that the buccal segment will move distally again following removal of the appliance, with opening of the contact area between upper lateral and first premolar. Particular attention should be paid to the axial inclination of the upper first premolar.

The mesial movement of the upper first premolar is often prevented by occlusal contact with lower teeth. Spot grinding may be necessary to relieve this.

In order that the appearance of the upper first premolar should be as near as possible to that of an upper canine, the tooth may require slight mesiopalatal rotation.

## REFERENCES

Farrant S. D. F. (1977) *Br. J. Orthod.* **4,** 5.
Griffiths P. J. T. (1970) *Trans. Br. Soc. Study Orthod.* **56,** 178.
Houston W. J. B. and Isaacson K. G. (1977) *Orthodontic Treatment with Removable Appliances.* Bristol, Wright.
Kettle M. A. (1958) *Dent. Pract. Dent. Rec.* **8,** 245.
Levason J. A. (1978) *Br. J. Orthod.* **5,** 5.
Plint D. A. (1961) *Dent. Pract. Dent. Rec.* **12,** 179.
Usiskin L. A. and Webb W. G. (1971) *Dent. Pract. Dent. Rec.* **21,** 437.
Wraith K. W. L. (1968) *Trans. Br. Soc. Study Orthod.* **55,** 47.

CHAPTER 10

# INCISOR ALIGNMENT

In this chapter we shall only describe the correction of incisor crowding and spacing. Proclination and retroclination of incisors, and overbite reduction, are considered in Chapter 11.

## INCISOR CROWDING

### The Nature of Incisor Crowding

When incisors occupy a space which would be inadequate to accommodate them if they were correctly aligned, the following abnormalities of tooth position are seen:
1. Labial or lingual displacement.
2. Rotational displacement.
3. Vertical displacement.
4. Abnormality of axial inclination.

In order to correct incisor crowding, space must therefore be made available. This will usually necessitate distal movement of the canines.

In many cases, if space is provided, there will be considerable spontaneous improvement in the position of teeth in the labial segments. This is often seen in the lower arch, where, following the extraction of lower first premolars, spontaneous distal movement of canines and improvement in incisor alignment occurs without the use of appliances. In other cases, particularly where there is considerable displacement of teeth in the labial segments, the amount of spontaneous improvement following upon the provision of space is minimal. Such displacements can be considered as not due solely to shortage of space, and appliances are required if these displacements are to be corrected.

The manner in which the required tooth movement can be achieved differs according to the kind of bracket that is employed, although the basic principles apply irrespective of the bracket system used.

The correction of incisor crowding will be described using edgewise brackets, Begg brackets and a system called 'Pin and Tube'.

### Edgewise Brackets

It is common practice to retract the canines before commencing alignment of the incisors. This often allows for some spontaneous improve-

91

ment in incisor crowding, and makes the subsequent banding of incisors easier.

When crowding is relatively mild it is possible to retract the canines and align the incisor simultaneously. Such a situation is often found in the lower arch. In the upper arch, however, such simultaneous tooth movement is usually only possible if additional anchorage is provided by extra-oral anchorage or intermaxillary traction. A discussion of anchorage considerations in these circumstances is to be found in Chapter 13.

*Plain Archwires*

Flexible plain archwires are useful in the early stages of the treatment of crowded incisors. They are effective in levelling of bracket height, correcting labial or lingual displacement, and, particularly when used in conjunction with brackets of considerable mesiodistal width (Siamese brackets), in producing rotation and uprighting.

The smaller the diameter of an archwire, the more flexible it is. High tensile wire of 0·30 mm diameter is sufficiently flexible in all planes to make it useful for initial aligning archwires. Partial engagement of the archwire is made when full engagement would result in excessive force being delivered or in permanent archwire deformation. After one or two appointments this archwire can be changed progressively to 0·35 mm and then to 0·40 mm diameter wire, incorporating vertical loops where required to increase flexibility. Full engagement of the archwire in the bracket channels should be obtained at an early stage of treatment in order to achieve the maximum control over tooth position. Final alignment is achieved using progressively thicker archwires, bent to ideal form. Where indicated, rectangular archwires

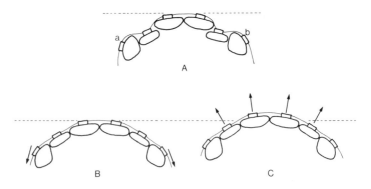

*Fig.* 10.1. Incisor alignment using small diameter plain archwire (*see text*).

may be used in the final stages, but their construction is difficult and should only be carried out by the experienced operator. The inflexibility of rectangular archwires makes them unsuitable for the correction of other than relatively minor tooth displacement, but ideally suited to precise repositioning and providing rigid retention.

Multistrand wire finds its main application in the early stages of incisor alignment. The wire is equally flexible in all planes, and does not need to be formed before being tied in.

When multistrand wire or small diameter plain round wires are used for initial alignment of incisors there is a tendency for them to produce incisor proclination (*Fig.* 10.1). Consider the span of archwire between points *a* and *b* (*Fig.* 10.1A). The archwire has been elastically deformed into the incisor brackets. Forces are applied to the teeth, which move as the span of archwire returns towards its passive configuration. The forces may be dissipated by labial movement of 2|2 without palatal movement of 1|1 or 3|3. If this is to occur, the archwire must slide distally through the canine brackets, or the canines must move distally with the archwire (*Fig.* 10.1B). In practice the movement of the archwire through the canine brackets will be restricted by friction (bracket binding), and the relatively large root area of the canines will minimize distal movement of 3|3. The usual result, therefore, is labial proclination of 21|12 and minimal distal movement of 3|3 (*Fig.* 10.1C). An improvement in alignment has been obtained at the expense of incisor proclination, which usually needs to be corrected at a later stage of treatment.

## Multilooped Archwires

Round-wire multilooped archwires are particularly useful for producing alignment of teeth in the labial segments. Canine retraction and incisor alignment can be carried out simultaneously. Because a relatively large number of teeth are being moved at the same time, there is a danger of excessive forward movement of posterior teeth, with resulting shortage of space for the alignment of canines and incisors. Such multiple tooth movements frequently require the use of additional anchorage, either from the opposing arch by the use of intermaxillary traction, or by using extra-oral traction.

Full engagement of the archwire in the bracket channels is achieved as soon as possible, and the teeth move with the archwire rather than sliding along the archwire.

The positioning of the vertical loops relative to the teeth is critical if maximum use of these archwires is to be realized.

In order to illustrate the way in which a multilooped archwire functions, the treatment of a crowded lower labial segment will be described.

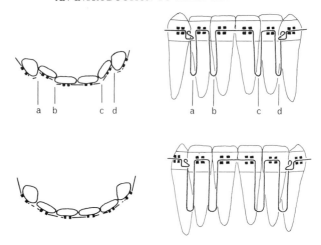

*Fig.* 10.2. Alignment of lower labial segment using multilooped archwire and edgewise brackets (*see text*).

*Fig.* 10.2 shows a crowded lower labial segment. The incisors are banded and carry Siamese edgewise brackets.

The functions of the various parts of the archwire will be considered:

THE HOOKS: These lie hard against the mesial aspect of the canine brackets, and the loops 'a' and 'd' are compressed so that a distally directed force is applied to the canines in order to move these teeth distally away from the incisors. The reaction to this force applied to the canines will tend to procline the incisors. This tendency can be offset by applying intramaxillary elastics from the archwire hook to the molar hook on each side. Alternatively, the canines can be tied back with elastic ligature or linked bracket elastics.

LOOPS 'a' and 'b' are compressed between the mesial of $\overline{3|}$ bracket and the distal of $\overline{1|}$ bracket. Thus as $\overline{3|}$ moves distally, $\overline{2|}$ moves distally relative to $\overline{1|}$, so providing space for $\overline{|2}$ to move labially.

LOOPS 'c' and 'd' provide flexibility for the rotation of $\overline{|2}$.

In this manner, alignment is readily achieved, but, because the width of the bracket restricts movement along the archwire, mesiodistal movement is only achieved by careful positioning and activation of the vertical loops.

Further adjustment of the vertical loops will allow overcorrection of rotation and labiolingual position to be achieved.

Vertical loops have their maximum effect of increasing flexibility in a plane at right angles to the plane in which they lie. The vertical looped archwire described above is therefore efficient in producing the labiolingual and rotational correction required. Vertical looped archwires are not sufficiently flexible to produce bracket levelling when the vertical discrepancy is marked. Under these conditions a plain archwire can be used initially (multistrand wire, for example) followed by a multilooped archwire incorporating horizontal loops (*see Fig.* 6.13).

## Practical Points

1. It is important to ensure that each horizontal section of the archwire can engage the appropriate bracket without the vertical arms of the loops contacting the teeth.

2. When the archwire is fully engaged the vertical loops must not press against the gingiva or protrude so far as to cause irritation to the lip. It should be borne in mind that as tooth movement proceeds the vertical loops may alter in their relationship to the gingival tissues. The archwire must be placed in the brackets and any alteration in the angulation of the vertical loops made before final engagement. Any adjustment of vertical loops must be made in both arms of the loop in order to preserve the 'flatness' of the archwire. Alteration of loop angulation is not permissible after final engagement of the archwire, because this will introduce unpredictable activation.

## Begg Brackets

The Begg bracket has minimal mesiodistal width and the archwire is a loose fit in the bracket channel. The following mechanical implications should be noted:

1. Because of the minimal mesiodistal width of the bracket, considerable overcorrection of those sections of the archwire being used to produce rotation is required (*Fig.* 10.3).

2. Because of the minimal mesiodistal width of the bracket, apical movements (uprighting and torqueing) are not possible without the use of accessory springs.

3. The loose fit of the archwire in the bracket channel allows tooth

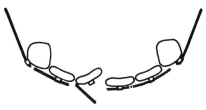

*Fig.* 10.3. Rotation of 1| using overcorrected looped section of archwire.

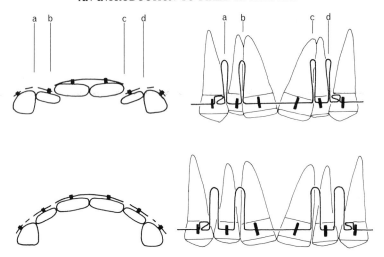

*Fig.* 10.4. Alignment of upper labial segment using multilooped archwire and Begg brackets (*see text*).

movement to occur by tipping, and movement of teeth along the archwire is facilitated.

Begg brackets may be used with both plain and multilooped round archwires. *Fig.* 10.4 shows a crowded upper labial segment. The teeth are banded and carry Begg brackets. The tooth movements required are:

'a'. Distal movement of 3|3. These teeth are mesially inclined and the appliance is designed to tip 3|3 distally.

'b'. Distal movement of 2|2.

'c'. Rotation of 2|2.

'd'. Uprighting of 1|1.

A round-wire mutilooped 0·40 mm diameter arch is prepared and pinned into the brackets. The function of the various parts of the archwire are as follows:

THE HOOKS: These lie hard against the mesial aspects of the canine brackets. When the arch is pinned in, the loops 'a', 'b', 'c', 'd', are compressed so that a distally directed force is applied to the canines. The canines will tip distally. The reaction to the force applied to the canines will tend to procline the incisors. Inter- or intramaxillary traction elastics applied to the hooks will offset this tendency.

LOOPS 'a' and 'b' are concerned with providing flexibility for the rotation and labial movement of 2|.

LOOPS 'b' and 'c' enable 2|2 to be moved distally away from 1|1.

The buccal spans of archwire running between the distal aspects of the canine brackets and the molar tubes are concerned with the control of intercanine width, and may incorporate anchorage bends (*see* Chapter 13).

The space required for the alignment of 2|2 is provided as canine retraction proceeds. When the canines have been moved far enough distally to provide enough for incisor alignment, further spontaneous distal tipping along the archwire is prevented by tying the canine brackets forwards onto the archwire hooks.

It should be noted that the multilooped archwire described has not corrected the apical position of 1|1. When Begg brackets are used, accessory springs are required to produce uprighting (*see* Chapter 6) or torqueing.

## *Begg Uprighting Springs*

Preformed uprighting springs are available for use with Begg brackets. They are inserted into the vertical pin-channel of the bracket, and the free end is bent into a hook which engages the archwire. The free arm is relatively short, but the helix provides flexibility.

These springs are very effective in producing apical movement, the loose fit of the archwire in the bracket allowing the tooth to pivot freely on the archwire. *Fig.* 10.5 illustrates the correction of the apical position of 1|1 using uprighting springs. Two reciprocal effects of the uprighting spring on the tooth must be taken into account:

1. The spring applies a force which will move the crown of the tooth in the opposite direction to that in which the apex is being moved. In the illustration (*Fig.* 10.5) the brackets on 1|1 must be

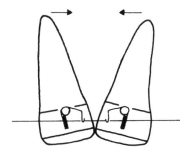

*Fig.* 10.5. Use of uprighting springs to correct the apical position of 1|1.
*Note:* The ligature tying 1|1 brackets together has been omitted for clarity.

ligated together, otherwise a maxillary median diastema will be produced.

2. The spring tends to move the tooth occlusally. Although the helix restricts this movement, the archwire may 'escape' between the helix and the band surface so that it no longer engages the bracket channel. In order to prevent this occlusal movement a ligature is placed round the archwire and the bracket. This ligature must not be so tight that the tooth is no longer free to pivot on the archwire.

Modified preformed uprighting springs are available which incorporate a locking pin, so ensuring that the archwire remains in the bracket channel without the need for a ligature to prevent it escaping.

### Begg Rotation Springs

Rotation springs may be attached to Begg brackets (*see Fig.* 6.16). The narrowness of the bracket channel allows the tooth to rotate on the archwire. Careful activation is required to ensure that the spring does not inadvertently act as an uprighting spring and produce tipping.

## Pin and Tube

The pin and tube appliance was described by Watkin (1933), and more recently by Leighton (1963), Clifford (1965), and Mills (1968). A brief description of its use is included in this chapter, but the reader is referred to the above references for a full description of the system.

### Construction

A limited number of teeth, usually incisors and molars only, are banded. The molars carry conventional round buccal tubes, but the anterior bands carry vertical boxes, similar to the female element of the McKeag lock, on their labial surfaces (*Fig.* 10.6). The archwire,

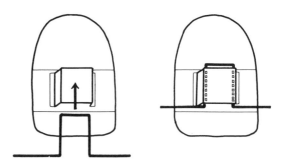

*Fig.* 10.6. Incisor attachment for pin and tube appliance.

usually 0·40 mm diameter wire, is bent in such a way as to form U-loops or 'pins' which fit firmly into the vertical slots. By suitable adjustment of the archwire tooth movement in any direction, including apical 'torque', can be achieved.

Inter- or intramaxillary elastics and extra-oral traction can be used in conjunction with a pin and tube appliance.

A description of the use of the pin and tube appliance for producing overjet reduction, including the principle of 'lever torque', can be found in Chapter 11.

## *Incisor Alignment with the Pin and Tube Appliance*

Because the teeth carrying vertical slots are 'locked' onto the archwire, it is possible to adjust the archwire in such a way as to produce tooth movement in any direction. The archwire spans between neighbouring teeth are formed into loops or helices in order that the archwire can be activated to produce the required tooth movement.

The archwire must be bent up and adjusted with the greatest care to make sure that it has not been activated in such a way as to produce unwanted tooth movement. The appliance is generally used to produce alignment of one or two anterior teeth only, because when more teeth are incorporated in the appliance archwire fabrication becomes extremely complicated.

DEROTATION OF A SINGLE TOOTH: Only the rotated tooth and the first permanent molars need be banded. The archwire is bent up, commencing at the pin, and the buccal sections are taken towards the sulcus in order to minimize archwire distortion under masticatory forces. The buccal arms are activated so that when the archwire is inserted a rotational force is applied to the incisor (*Fig.* 10.7B).

In many cases a tooth may be so severely rotated that it becomes difficult to carry the archwire into the most palatally displaced corner of the tooth. In such cases the rotation can be commenced by using an archwire with a single buccal arm, which acts as a whip (*Fig.* 10.7A).

UPRIGHTING A SINGLE TOOTH: The principle is the same as that for producing rotation, except that in this case one buccal arm is activated in a gingival direction and the other in an occlusal direction (*Fig.* 10.7C).

By suitable activation, both uprighting and rotation can be carried out at the same time. Unless great attention is given to archwire adjustment, unwanted rotational or uprighting forces can inadvertently be applied.

ALIGNMENT OF CENTRAL INCISORS: When a maxillary diastema is to be closed the pin and tube appliance may be of advantage since it enables the incisors to be moved together bodily. 'Overcorrection' of the apical position of the incisors, as well as rotation, can be achieved. The archwire span between the central incisors carries vertical loops and helices, and care must be taken to ensure that the archwire does not irritate the labial fraenum (*Fig.* 10.8).

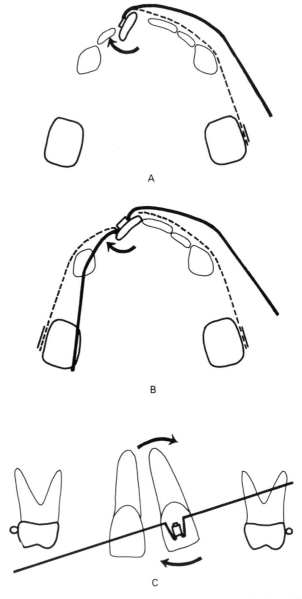

*Fig.* 10.7. Pin and tube mechanisms used to align a single incisor. A, B, Correction of a rotated incisor. C, Archwire activated to upright ⌊1.

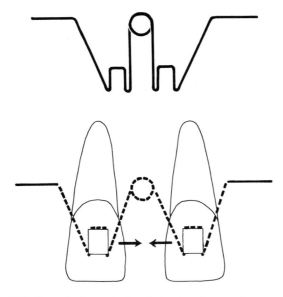

*Fig.* 10.8. Pin and tube mechanism designed to close maxillary median diastema.

## SPACE CLOSURE

Spacing in the incisor region is liable to reappear following space closure unless the following principles are observed:

1. Complete closure of the space.
2. Root paralleling.
3. Establishment of intact contact points in the arch.

### Complete Closure of the Space

ELASTICS: Elastic ligature, or latex elastics, can be used to produce space closure. Elastic ligature requires replacement at each visit. Latex elastics can be attached by the patient to long Begg pins which have been formed into hooks. Space closure will occur by tipping if Begg brackets have been used.

With edgewise brackets, linked bracket elastics are effective for producing space closure. The relatively wide brackets must slide along the archwire as the teeth move under the influence of the elastic traction, and less tipping is to be expected than when Begg brackets are used.

MULTILOOPED ARCHWIRES: Vertical loops can be used (*Fig.* 10.9) to close incisor spacing. It is often advantageous to incorporate a helix in the loop to provide more flexibility. When vertical loops are used with

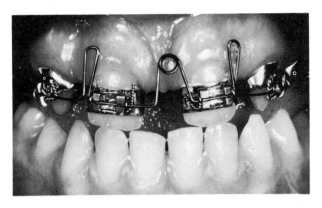

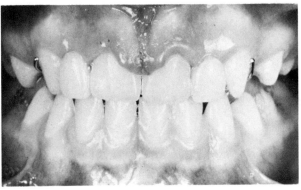

*Fig.* 10.9. A, Vertical loops and helix used to close diastema between 1|1. B, After removal of fixed appliance and insertion of removable prosthesis to replace 2|2.

wide brackets the arch can be adjusted to minimize tipping as the space is closed. There is a danger that the incisors may rotate during space closure, and the arch must be activated to prevent this.

PIN AND TUBE: A pin and tube appliance is particularly useful for the closure of a single space in the incisor region because the teeth can be moved bodily together. Rotations can be corrected at the same time.

### Root Paralleling
When the incisor spacing has been completely eliminated by one of the methods described in the previous section, attention must be paid to the correction of apical position. If elastics have been used to move teeth along the archwire into contact, the teeth will have tipped together. Unless they are uprighted, the spaces are liable to reopen as the teeth relapse towards their initial inclination.

The incisor crowns must first be firmly tied together in order that the spaces do not reopen when the uprighting mechanism is applied.

If Begg brackets have been used uprighting springs are applied to correct apical position.

If wide brackets are used a multilooped section can be activated to produce uprighting, care being taken to ensure that the archwire does not rotate in the brackets and cause rotation of the teeth.

The apical positions should be overcorrected as a safeguard against reopening of the spaces and maintained with an archwire incorporating bayonet offsets. A radiographic check of apical position following uprighting is desirable.

## Establishment of Intact Contact Points

In order to reduce the possibility of reopening of incisor spaces it is necessary to move the buccal segments and canines forwards so that no spacing remains in the arch. In some cases, particularly where spacing is due to missing or extracted teeth, a prosthesis may be fitted following tooth alignment, which will help to restore intact contact points.

When teeth in the buccal segments are moved forwards it is again important to upright them, to reduce the possibility of relapse (*see* Chapter 9). At band removal, small spaces will be left between the contact points owing to the thickness of the band material. A removable appliance should be fitted as soon as possible after band removal and activated to eliminate completely these band spaces.

## SEVERELY DISPLACED INCISORS

It is sometimes necessary to realign an upper incisor which has failed to erupt to its correct level. Such teeth are frequently rotated, with their apices considerably displaced. The preliminary stage of treatment involves movement of adjacent teeth in order to provide sufficient space for the realignment. The displacement is usually so severe that it is not practicable to construct an archwire to begin realignment of the displaced incisor. Under these circumstances a rigid base archwire is attached to the remaining teeth, which should ideally carry edgewise brackets. Elastic traction can then be applied from the archwire to the displaced tooth. The method of attachment of the elastic traction to the displaced tooth will depend upon the local conditions. Sometimes it is possible to cement a band with suitable attachment. Alternatively a direct-bonded attachment can be used. In either case the location of the point of attachment of the elastic, and the direction of pull, must be considered in order to move the tooth in the correct direction.

The greater part of the required occlusal movement can be achieved in this way. Eventually the tooth will be in such a position that it can be banded conventionally, and an edgewise bracket used. At this stage an accessory plain multistrand archwire can be applied to continue the correction, the base archwire remaining in position. As the displaced incisor moves near to its final position, the base and accessory archwires are discarded and a multilooped archwire incorporating horizontal loops is used, care being taken over apical, rotational, and occlusal correction.

## SECTIONAL ARCHES FOR INCISOR ALIGNMENT

Sectional arches are used for incisor alignment when the treatment is limited to alignment of the labial segment, without alteration of the overbite or overjet. They are used, therefore, for space closure following the extraction of an incisor, for the closure of median diastema, and for the correction of incisor position when sufficient space for alignment is present.

The principles of reciprocal anchorage apply when sectional arches are used, and it is usually advisable to band and incorporate the canines in the appliance. In this way more control over the movement of incisors is obtained.

Rectangular wire engaging edgewise brackets can be used. Sectional alignment mechanisms can also be made from round wire, engaging edgewise brackets, or the vertical tubes of the pin and tube appliance.

Mesiodistal and buccolingual movements may be produced by a multilooped sectional archwire. Elastics can be used for space closure.

## CENTRE LINE CORRECTION

It may be necessary during treatment to move the upper centre line relative to the lower, perhaps to produce coincidence of the two centre lines.

The following methods can be used to produce alteration of centre line:

1. Individual tooth movement. Incisors are moved individually along the archwire in a lateral direction using elastics, elastic ligature, or linked bracket elastics.

2. Anterior cross-elastic. An elastic stretched between archwire hooks lying, for instance, mesial to 3⌋ and mesial to ⌈3 will produce alteration in the relative position of upper and lower centre lines.

3. Vertical loops. An archwire carrying vertical loops placed between the canines and lateral incisors can be activated in such a way that the position of the centre line is changed. One of the two loops is adjusted to be 'compressed' between the canine and lateral in-

cisor brackets and the other adjusted to be 'expanded' when the archwire is tied in.

4. The use of unilateral inter- or intramaxillary traction can produce changes in centre line position.

5. If a centre line shift has become associated with tipping of incisors, then uprighting springs can sometimes be used to move the centre line and upright the incisors simultaneously. The incisor crowns are allowed to move along the archwire under the influence of the uprighting spring.

## REFERENCES

Clifford E. J. S. (1965) *Trans. Br. Soc. Study Orthod. Dent Pract. Dent. Rec.* **16,** 35.

Leighton B. C. (1963) *Trans. Br. Soc. Orthodont.* 106.

Mills J. R. E. (1968) *Dent. Prac. Dent. Rec.* **18,** 185.

Mills J. R. E. (1968) *Trans. Br. Soc. Study. Orthod.* **55,** 135.

Watkin H. G. (1933) *Trans. Br. Soc. Orthodont.* 'Pin and tube appliances'.

# CHAPTER 11

# OVERBITE AND OVERJET

Reduction of overjet is achieved in most cases by movement of the upper incisor crowns in a palatal direction. Labial movement of the lower incisor crowns as an aid to overjet reduction should usually be avoided, because the lower incisors may be brought into an unstable position from which they are liable to relapse following the removal of appliances.

When the overbite is increased, movement of the upper incisor crowns in a palatal direction may be prevented by the position of the lower incisor crowns. Without reduction of overbite the palatal surfaces of the upper incisor crowns meet the lower incisors before the overjet is adequately reduced (*Fig.* 11.1).

Overbite and overjet control are thus closely interdependent.

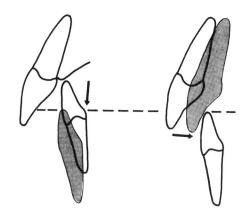

*Fig.* 11.1. Overbite reduction prior to overjet reduction.

## OVERBITE REDUCTION

Two possibilities exist for 'depressing' the lower incisors:

TRUE DEPRESSION: This involves depressing the lower incisors axially into the alveolus so that the distance between the lower border of the mandible and the incisal edges decreases. True depression is very difficult to achieve.

RELATIVE DEPRESSION: The lower incisor vertical development is arrested, while the buccal segments continue to develop vertically; this means that the mandibular base is moved away from the maxillary base in the sagittal plane. This is associated with an increase in the maxillary-mandibular planes angle, which is liable to revert towards its former value after treatment.

Both relative and true depression may occur together when a fixed appliance is used.

Overbite is easier to reduce in the young patient than in the adult, presumably because in the adult growth changes are complete. Overbite reduction is also reputed to be more difficult in patients with a low anterior facial height.

## Methods of Reducing Overbite

### Bite Planes

Increased overbites are readily reduced by the use of a flat anterior bite plane incorporated in an upper removable appliance. The bite plane will produce relative depression of the incisors. Except when removed for cleaning, the appliance should be worn full time. With the appliance in place, the buccal segments should be separated by a small amount (1–2 mm). As the lower incisors are 'depressed', the bite plane is increased in depth by the addition of cold cure acrylic to the surface which occludes with the lower incisors, in order to maintain buccal segment separation.

An increase in overjet is sometimes seen when such appliances are worn, due to the appliance 'settling in' to the palatal mucosa and bearing against the upper incisors. An increase in the maxillary-mandibular planes angle, resulting from the use of a bite plane, has the effect of increasing the severity of a Class II malocclusion (*see* p. 63).

Bite planes can be used in the early stages of treatment in cases which will eventually require fixed appliances. The upper removable appliance carrying the bite plane may, for example, incorporate springs to commence canine retraction. The bite plane should be designed not to cause alteration of the lower incisor axial inclination.

Following the use of a bite plane, a lower fixed appliance will be required to maintain the overbite reduction which has been achieved, in order that the overjet can be reduced with a fixed appliance.

### Archwires for Overbite Reduction

PLAIN ARCHWIRES: Increased overbites are often associated with an exaggerated curve of Spee, and a plain archwire lying in the molar tubes rests passively well below the level of the incisor band brackets. The effect of inserting such a plain archwire is to produce a reduction of the overbite, principally by relative depression of the lower incisors, although some intrusion of the incisors may occur. Archwires of progressively increasing diameters are used, the final archwires being constructed with a reverse curve of Spee.

Archwires which are very flexible, such as multistrand archwires or multilooped archwires, are not effective in producing overbite reduction, and initial alignment of the lower arch must be achieved before overbite reduction can be completed.

ANCHORAGE BENDS: These are placed just mesial to the molar tubes and are activated so that an archwire of 0·40 mm lies between 10–15 mm below the level of the lower incisor brackets. Anchorage bends of this kind are most effective when the archwire is not engaged in the premolar brackets. The size of anchorage bend that is used will depend upon the curve of Spee, but the bend should not exceed 30° (see p. 121).

The reciprocal force to that which 'depresses' the lower incisors produces a distal tipping and elevation of the lower molars. Class II intermaxillary traction is often used in conjunction with anchorage bends, and aids in overbite reduction by imparting a vertical component of force to the lower molars.

It should be noted that anchorage bends will sometimes produce proclination of the lower incisors, especially in cases where the lower incisors are proclined before treatment.

LOOPED ARCHWIRES: An archwire incorporating horizontal loops in the incisor region will provide sufficient flexibility for levelling and hence overbite reduction.

ACCESSORY ARCHWIRES: These are designed to engage the molar tubes and lower incisors only, whilst buccal segment tooth position is controlled by sectional archwires: this necessitates the use of additional lower molar buccal tubes. These archwires are activated gingivally, and the long unsupported buccal section, often incorporating a helix, increases the flexibility of these archwires in the vertical plane.

UPPER ARCH: When movement of the upper incisors towards the maxillary base is required to produce a stable interincisal relationship, anchorage bends may be used in the upper arch. This movement can be aided by the use of high-pull headgear and J hooks, engaged on the anterior part of the upper archwire.

## OVERJET REDUCTION

The factors which determine the stability of the incisor relationship, and aesthetic considerations, will decide the 'ideal' final position of the upper incisors.

The type of mechanism used will determine the movement of the upper incisors which is produced.

A palatally directed force applied by point contact to the labial surfaces of the upper incisors produces tipping in a palatal direction, and hence reduction of overjet. This is the sort of movement produced by upper removable appliances when used to reduce an overjet.

It is not possible at the present time to predict accurately the translation in position of an upper incisor under the influence of a palatally directed tipping force. A variable amount of labial movement of the upper incisor apices is produced. In some cases labial movement of the incisor apex during overjet reduction is desirable, or at least produces an adequate and stable interincisal relationship. In other cases, however, any labial movement of the upper incisor apices during overjet reduction is undesirable; and sometimes it is necessary to move the upper incisor apices in a palatal direction compared with their pretreatment position. When appliances are used to move incisor apices intentionally either buccally or lingually, the movement is referred to as 'torqueing'. When an increased overjet is the result of a marked Class II skeletal pattern, the upper incisors may be at an average axial inclination to the maxillary plane. If simple tipping with removable appliances is used to reduce the overjet in these cases, the upper incisors will be severely retroclined at the completion of overjet reduction, with an unsatisfactory appearance and the possibility of a traumatic overbite. Palatal apical torque of the incisors is indicated in these cases, resulting in a better appearance and incisor relationship (*Fig.* 11.2).

The methods used for reducing an overjet will be discussed under the following headings:

1. Overjet reduction by tipping of upper incisors.
2. Overjet reduction with apical control.

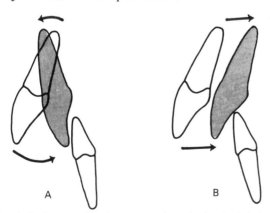

*Fig.* 11.2. A comparison between overjet reduction by (A) tipping the upper incisor crowns distally and (B) retraction of upper incisors by bodily movement.

## Overjet Reduction by Tipping of the Upper Incisors

If a palatally directed force is delivered to the labial surfaces of the incisors by means of an archwire of circular cross-section running through the brackets, the incisor crowns are moved in a palatal direction. Since the round archwire is free to rotate in the brackets, there is no control of the movement of the incisor apices in a labiopalatal direction. Whether or not apical movement is produced will depend upon the centre, or centres, of rotation produced in the incisors by the applied force. The mechanism will at any rate not induce movement of the apices in a palatal direction.

When the canines are retracted before overjet reduction is commenced they must be tied back to the molars, to prevent relapse of their position during overjet reduction. Prior to commencing overjet reduction, the incisors must be well aligned and all spaces between the incisors closed.

CLOSING LOOPS: For overjet reduction an archwire with closing loops just distal to the laterals is constructed, and is activated by pulling the archwire through the molar tubes and turning it down (*Fig.* 11.3). An

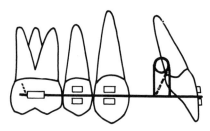

*Fig.* 11.3. Archwire, 0·40 mm, for overjet reduction using closing loops.

alternative method of activation is by means of a tie-back ligature attached to a traction hook.

If there is a chance of the posterior teeth moving too far forward, as a reaction to the activation of the closing loops during overjet reduction, the anchorage must be reinforced by means of Class II intermaxillary traction elastics or extra-oral traction.

EXTRA-ORAL TRACTION: When overjet reduction is achieved by means of extra-oral traction applied to J hooks in the anterior section of the upper archwire, the movement is not dependent upon intra-oral anchorage. In addition, the translation in position of the upper incisors can be influenced by alteration of the direction of pull.

ELASTIC TRACTION: Using a Johnson twin-wire arch an overjet can be reduced with elastic inter- or intramaxillary traction. The end tubes

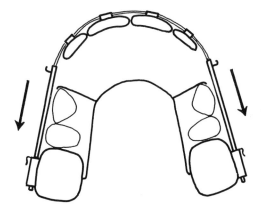

*Fig.* 11.4. Twin-wire arch for overjet reduction, using intramaxillary elastic traction.

must be free-sliding in the molar tubes, and the elastic is applied to hooks on the end tubes (*Fig.* 11.4).

A similar principle can be employed with an archwire which is bent with traction hooks distal to the lateral incisors. If, in order to ensure that this archwire is free-sliding in the buccal segments, the canines are not attached, there is a long unsupported section of wire which is liable to distortion (*Fig.* 11.5). If the upper labial segment is crowded, vertical loops can be incorporated between the incisors so that alignment and overjet reduction can be carried out simultaneously.

*Lever Torque*

The principle of lever torque is worthy of particular mention, as it enables the upper incisor crowns to be moved in a palatal direction

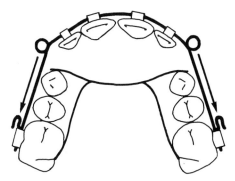

*Fig.* 11.5. Archwire, 0·40 mm, for ovejet reduction, using elastic traction to the archwire hooks.

111

without a mesially directed force being applied to the upper molars. The upper incisor bands carry the vertical slots which are used in the Watkin pin and tube appliance. The molar bands carry horizontal buccal tubes. The archwire is usually constructed from 0·45 mm round stainless-steel high tensile wire, inserted into the incisor attachments (*see Fig*. 10.6). The distal ends of the archwire lie passively

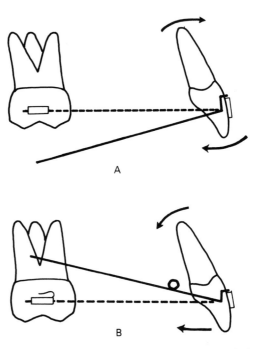

*Fig*. 11.6. Pin and tube appliance. A, Overjet reduction by tipping of the incisors. B, Overjet reduction with intramaxillary elastic traction used to prevent labial movement of the upper incisor apices.

about 1 cm below the buccal tubes. When the archwire is fully engaged the action is to tip the crowns palatally and the apices labially. Providing the archwire is free to slide distally through the molar tubes, the incisors will be 'uprighted' (*Fig*. 11.6A). It is the movement of the upper incisor apices in a labial direction which makes the mechanism unsuitable for the reduction of overjet in the majority of cases. It should be noticed, however, that the only reciprocal action on the molar teeth is to extrude them, and in practice this produces no noticeable effect.

It is possible to adapt the principle of lever torque in such a way as to prevent labial movement of the upper incisor apices during overjet reduction. *Fig.* 11.6B shows an archwire inserted into the incisor attachments. The distal ends of the archwire lie passively above the molar tubes. When the arch is inserted it tends to move the upper incisor apices palatally and the crowns labially. Intramaxillary traction is applied, between archwire hooks and hooks on the molar bands, in order to produce movement of the incisor crowns in a palatal direction. There is thus a reciprocal, mesially directed force applied to the molars, and extra-oral traction may well be required to prevent these teeth moving too far forward.

## *Overjet Reduction with Apical Control*

When reducing overjets with fixed appliances it is sometimes desirable to reduce the overjet by tipping of the incisors first, and then to correct the axial inclination of the incisors by palatal root torque. Alternatively, the incisors may be retracted bodily.

A considerable amount of anchorage is required for palatal movement of incisor apices, and bodily retraction of incisors necessitates the use of relatively high forces. Reinforcement of anchorage by extra-oral force, by Class II intermaxillary traction, or a combination of both, is almost invariably necessary.

Torqueing archwires tend to cause an expansion of intermolar width, and compensating bends must be made to contract the archwire or the intermolar width stabilized by means of a palatal or lingual arch.

### *Round Archwires*

In order to produce palatal apical movement of incisors, a force couple must be applied to the crown of the tooth. With round archwires this is achieved by means of a two-point contact on the labial face of the tooth. The reciprocal of a palatally directed force applied by the torqueing mechanism to the incisor apex is a labially directed force applied to the bracket. Torqueing mechanisms therefore produce an increase in overjet unless inter- or intramaxillary or extra-oral traction is used.

TORQUEING SPURS: These are vertical loops in the archwire which contact the labial surface of the incisor near the gingival margin. The angulation of the spur is adjusted so that they deliver a palatally directed force to the roots of the incisors. *Fig.* 11.7A shows an archwire of 0·45 mm diameter carrying vertical torqueing spurs, used with Siamese edgewise brackets. *Fig.* 11.7B shows the Begg type of torqueing spurs, usually made as an auxiliary in wire of 0·35 mm diameter with a 0·5 mm base archwire.

WOUND-ON TORQUEING AUXILIARY: The auxiliary is constructed of

113

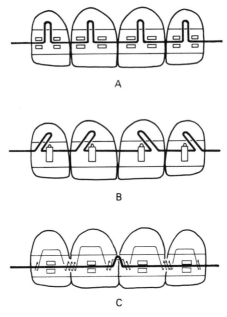

*Fig.* 11.7. Round-wire torqueing mechanisms. A, Vertical torqueing spurs for use with Siamese edgewise brackets. B, Begg-type torqueing spurs. C, Wound-on torqueing auxiliary.

0·35 mm diameter high-tensile wire and is supported on the base archwire, which is 0·5 mm diameter wire (*Fig.* 11.8). The wound-on auxiliary is sufficiently flexible to produce considerable movement of the apices in a palatal direction without requiring reactivation. The force it delivers is readily controlled and each section is individually adjustable. The relative inflexibility of the base archwire provides maximum control of molar position and restricts labial movement of the crowns of the incisors. This auxiliary is used to move the apices of the incisors in a palatal direction when the overjet has been reduced. It is of particular use when a considerable amount of palatal movement of upper incisor apices is required.

*Rectangular Archwires*
The advantage of rectangular archwires in the control of apical position is that the close fit of a rectangular archwire in the bracket slot enables buccopalatal movement of the apices to be achieved by torsion of the archwire. Torqueing auxiliaries are therefore not necessary. Because of the relative inflexibility of rectangular archwires, frequent reactivation of the archwire is required to increase the amount of root

114

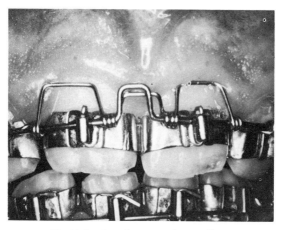

*Fig.* 11.8. Wound-on torqueing auxiliary.

torque. To increase the flexibility, helices may be incorporated in the archwire distal to the lateral incisors. A torqueing archwire may also be constructed with helices just anterior to the molar tubes with the archwire clear of the brackets of the premolars and canines, which have to be controlled with separate sectional archwires. This archwire is more flexible than a plane rectangular wire and requires less reactivation.

CLOSING LOOPS: A rectangular archwire with closing loops distal to the lateral incisors can be used to reduce an overjet and will control the incisor apical position. The mechanics of a closing loop archwire are such that the amount of palatal root torque that is applied to the incisors is at its maximum when the loops have just been activated, but as the loops close the torque is reduced. This, unfortunately, limits the amount of torque that can be applied.

FREE-SLIDING ARCHWIRE: A rectangular archwire which is not engaged in brackets in the buccal segments and is free to slide through buccal tubes on the molars can be used to reduce an overjet bodily. A combination of extra-oral anchorage applied by J hooks to the anterior part of the archwire, and intramaxillary elastic traction would provide the retraction force. If necessary, the amount of torque could be increased as the overjet is reduced.

### Reverse Torque

This is a term applied to the movement of incisor apices in a labial direction. When using round-wire arches two-point contact is arranged so that one point as before is situated in the bracket channel, whereas the second point is now nearer to the incisal edge than the bracket channel. Such a mechanism applied to upper incisors will tend to move the crowns palatally at the expense of forward movement of the apices.

Reverse torque is sometimes applied to lower incisors to make them more resistant to proclination. This mechanism tends to move their apices labially and their crowns lingually. It can also be applied by means of rectangular archwires.

## OVERBITE AND OVERJET IN CLASS III INCISOR RELATIONSHIPS

The treatment of these cases presents special problems. Where there is a postural element, a small 'reversed' overjet and an increased overbite, the prognosis for correcting the incisor relationship is favourable. Cases with a severe Class III dental base relationship, a 'reversed' overjet, and no postural element carry a poor prognosis for producing a stable result with the upper incisors labial to the lower incisors. In some cases orthodontic treatment is limited to aligning both arches individually and accepting their Class III relationship.

The principles of correcting Class III incisor relationship by orthodontic means are:

1. Correction of the anteroposterior aspect of the incisor relationship mainly by proclination of the upper incisors, but also, to a lesser extent, by obtaining as much lower incisor retroclination as is compatible with stability.

2. Establishment of an adequate degree of overbite to maintain the upper incisors in their correct position.

3. Completion of the case by closing extraction spaces in the upper arch so that the buccal segments support the labial segment in its forward position. This is not so important in cases completed with an adequate degree of overbite, but it may provide the essential support in those cases where overbite is minimal.

In cases in which there is a considerable amount of 'reversed' overbite an upper removable appliance incorporating buccal overlays (only just sufficiently thick to allow proclination of the upper incisors) is useful for the short period required to move the upper incisors over the bite.

The anchorage for proclination of the upper incisors is provided by the buccal segments, which therefore may be moved distally. Bearing in mind the desirability of completing treatment in the upper arch with intact contact points, distal movement of the upper buccal segments may be a factor which detracts from the final stability of the incisor relationship. Class III traction tends to prevent distal movement of the upper buccal segments. In addition, Class III traction, perhaps in conjunction with intramaxillary traction in the lower arch, aids retroclination of the lower incisors.

Proclination of the upper incisors is best achieved by applying a labially directed force to their labial surfaces. The archwire must be carefully checked to see that it does not inadvertently deliver an intrusive force to the upper incisors, so tending to reduce the overbite. Compressed coils in the buccal segments can be used to deliver the proclining force, with the buccal span of archwire 'free-sliding' through the molar tubes.

If a multilooped archwire is used, teeth in the buccal segments can be firmly attached to the archwire because the buccal span of archwire is not free-sliding through the brackets. Correction of rotation and buccopalatal position of teeth in the buccal segments can then be effected at the same time as incisor proclination.

Some space to relieve crowding in Class III cases is obtained by proclination of the upper incisors. This fact, and the desirability of completing the upper arch with intact contact points, makes distal movement of upper buccal segments without extractions near the front of the arch a useful treatment plan for some Class III cases. Extra-oral traction is used to move the upper buccal segments distally, usually by its application to first molar bands. Extra-oral traction may increase the maxillary-mandibular planes angle, as discussed previously, and thus cause a reduction in overbite, which is frequently undesirable in Class III cases. Care must be taken to be sure that the extra-oral arch does not bear against the upper incisors.

Retroclination of the lower incisors is achieved by the use of Class III traction and intramaxillary traction in the lower arch. If there is only a small amount of space available in the lower arch, intramaxillary traction should not be used.

Intramaxillary traction is applied in the lower arch either by an active archwire with closing loops distal to the lower canines or by means of latex elastics running between molar hooks and hooks mesial to the canines. If the lower canines must be moved distally away from the incisors to relieve crowding, the hooks should lie hard against the mesial of the canine brackets. A multilooped labial section will aid incisor alignment.

Class III traction is applied to latex elastics running from hooks lying in front of the lower canines to hooks on the upper molar bands. This force can be transmitted to the upper archwire by means of stops in the arch bent to contact the mesial of the upper molar tubes.

In some Class III cases the degree of overbite when the upper incisors have been moved forward of the lower incisors is minimal. During treatment, care should be taken not to apply inadvertently intrusive forces to the upper (or lower) incisors. In those cases where the overbite is minimal the use of vertical elastics will create an overbite by 'elevation' of the incisors. Unfortunately, a considerable amount of this overbite may disappear following treatment. The small amount gained, however, may be critical to the stability of the treated case.

## REFERENCES

Clifford E. J. S. (1965) *Trans. Br. Soc. Study Orthod.* 29.
Haack D. C. (1963) *Am. J. Orthod.* **49,** 330.
Mills J. R. E. (1968) *Trans. Br. Soc. Study Orthod.* **55,** 135.
Sims M. R. (1971) *Am. J. Orthod.* **59,** 456.

## CHAPTER 12

# MOLAR CONTROL

During fixed-appliance treatment, adverse movement of the molars is often encountered. It is important to be aware of the possible complications of molar movement in order that action can be taken at each stage of treatment to correct or prevent these faults.

The unwanted movements which may arise are related to the forces applied to the molars by the fixed-appliance system.

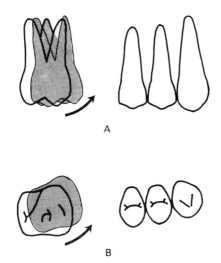

*Fig.* 12.1. Spontaneous forward movement of upper molars results in (A) mesial tipping and (B) mesiopalatal rotation.

### Forward Movement

Unwanted forward movement of molars may occur when they are used to provide anchorage for the distal movement of anterior teeth. The forward movement which is seen in these circumstances may well simulate the movement which occurs when molars move forward spontaneously—for example, following the early loss of deciduous molars or first permanent molars. Incorrect archwire form or faulty application of inter- or intramaxillary elastics may exaggerate these movements.

The results of spontaneous forward movement of molars differ in the upper and lower arches:

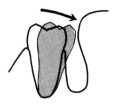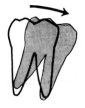

*Fig.* 12.2. Spontaneous forward movement of lower molars results in (A) lingual roll and (B) mesial tipping.

UPPER MOLARS (*Fig.* 12.1): As upper molars move forward they usually tip mesially and rotate mesiopalatally around their palatal roots.

LOWER MOLARS (*Fig.* 12.2): When lower molars move forward they usually tip mesially to a much greater extent than is seen in the case of upper molars. They also roll lingually.

*Expansion and Contraction*

Molar cross-bite may be present at the commencement of treatment, but in addition a fixed appliance may cause unwanted buccal or lingual movement of upper and lower molars.

An 0·40 or 0·45 mm diameter archwire with a discrepancy of 4–5 mm in the intermolar distance will not cause much immediate effect, especially if the cuspal relationship of the upper and lower molars restricts such movement. If throughout treatment each successive archwire is expanded, an increase in intermolar width may eventually be produced. Reference models provide a very useful record of the original intermolar width.

Archwires designed to produce apical torque of incisors may produce buccal expansion of the molars. The reason for this is that the torqueing spurs, or auxiliary, when passive, form an arc of a smaller radius than the radius of curvature of the labial segment. When the archwire is tied in to the brackets the spurs are forced into a wider arc. This deformation of the archwire is transmitted to the buccal segments as expansion. To counteract this a heavy base archwire is used, e.g., 0·50 mm diameter, and the archwire is made with a reduced inter-molar width. Correction of premolar rotation may also apply a buccal or lingual force to the archwire.

## METHODS OF MOLAR CONTROL

The means of molar control which are available are:

1. Archwire form.
2. Elastics.

3. Extra-oral traction.
4. Palatal and lingual arches.

In many cases molars will present at the beginning of treatment in an undesirable position. The mechanisms described are also applicable to the correction of such problems.

### Archwire Form

Forward movement of molars is inhibited by *anchorage bends*. These are bends at approximately 30° to the occlusal plane, and are placed in the archwire just mesial to the molars (*Fig.* 12.3A). They prevent

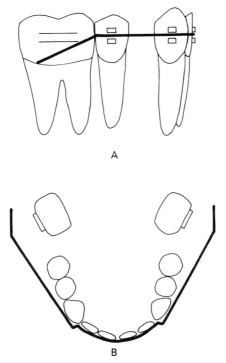

A

B

*Fig.* 12.3. A, Anchorage bend in a lower 0·40 or 0·45 mm diameter archwire. B, Archwire, 0·40 mm, to correct mesiolingual roll of 7|7. The archwire is expanded, and incorporates 'toe-in' bends.

forward tipping of the molars. If they are excessive the molars may be tipped distally, the mesial marginal ridge elevated, and the apices brought forward. If this has happened, when the appliance is removed the molar will tilt forward again and may cause recurrence of anterior crowding. A complication of using anchorage bends is that they may rotate in the molar tube and, instead of acting in the vertical plane, become effective in the horizontal plane, tending to move the distal of the molar buccally or lingually. To guard against this, check that the archwire lies in the 12 o'clock position in the molar tube when it is fully tied in.

Mesiolingual rotation is prevented by bends just in front of the molars, made in the horizontal plane again at about an angle of 30° to the buccal span of the archwire. These are called 'toe-in' bends and their effect is to rotate the molar mesiobuccally (*Fig.* 12.3B). Mesiolingual roll of lower molars (especially lower second molars) is corrected by a combination of anchorage bend and toe-in bend. It is also important to have the archwire expanded across the intermolar width by about 1 cm.

Correct positioning of the molar tubes is essential. If the tube is not at right angles to the long axis of the tooth or not parallel to the mesiodistal axis, rotation or tipping of the molar will be encouraged.

### *Elastics*

Intra- and intermaxillary elastic traction can, if incorrectly applied, cause deterioration of molar position. Class II traction in particular, if it is applied over the distal end of a buccal tube, will encourage tipping and rotation of a molar (*Fig.* 12.4). Intramaxillary traction similarly applied may cause rotation. If the elastic is hooked onto the archwire itself, as it projects through the distal end of the molar tube, the force may cause distortion of the archwire and rotation of the molar.

The ideal position for the attachment of elastics is to a mesial hook, as this will minimize the rotational effect of forward movement and counteract tipping. Some preformed buccal tubes which are now available have a slot which passes forwards from the distal end of the tube. This means that the point of application of the elastic force is about the midpoint of the buccal surface of the molar.

In the lower arch one of the best ways of preventing adverse movement is by the use of mesiolingual hooks, or buttons, for the application of Class II traction. This has the combined effect of pulling the mesiolingual aspect of the tooth buccally and vertically, thus preventing both rotation and tipping of the tooth. It is sometimes useful to apply the elastics alternately to the lingual and buccal aspects of the molars, for example, buccal by day and lingual by night.

### *Molar Cross-bite*

When a cross-bite is present it is usually best to correct it, if possible, at an early stage of treatment. The opposing molars concerned are banded and a hook fitted lingually on the tooth which is displaced lingually, and buccally on the other molar. These two hooks are joined

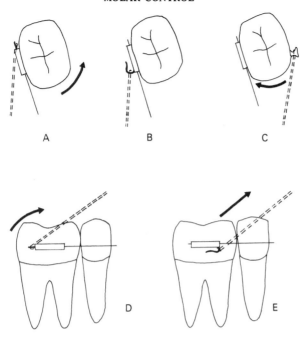

*Fig.* 12.4. The effect of Class II elastic traction applied to 6|6. A, The unwanted rotational force if the elastic is applied over the distal end of the archwire. B, Attachment to a mesiobuccal hook reduces unwanted rotation. C, Any tendency to mesiolingual roll is counteracted by attaching the Class II elastics to a mesiolingual button. D, Attachment of Class II elastics over the distal end of the archwire encourages unwanted tipping of the molar. E, Attachment of Class II elastics to a mesiobuccal hook restricts mesial tipping.

by an elastic—as small an elastic as the patient can manage—to offer a large force to the molars (*Fig.* 12.5). Small elastics worn double are very useful for this movement.

Cross-elastics may be used during treatment to correct any tendency to cross-bite that may arise.

### Extra-oral Traction

Extra-oral traction, when applied to upper first molar bands, is useful for correcting upper molar position. It can prevent forward movement of molars, and in cases where this has already occurred can, together with distal movement of these teeth, derotate and upright them.

It is possible also to expand or contract the intermolar width by simple adjustment of the inner arch of the extra-oral bow.

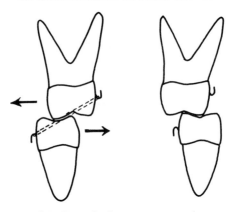

*Fig.* 12.5. Cross-elastics to correct a molar cross-bite.

## *Palatal and Lingual Arches*

Palatal and lingual arches are particularly useful for producing contraction or expansion of intermolar width. An appreciable force is required for this movement and the force exerted by an 0·40 or 0·45 mm diameter buccal arch is inadequate for producing deliberate contraction or expansion. Palatal and lingual arches can also be activated to produce a limited amount of molar rotation or uprighting.

## FIRST MOLAR EXTRACTIONS

### *Lower Molars*

From an orthodontic point of view the late extraction of lower first molars is undesirable. There is little spontaneous relief of lower incisor crowding, and the second molars will roll lingually as they move forward, in most cases not making satisfactory contact with the second premolar. Many malocclusions which could otherwise have been treated quite simply are complicated by the enforced loss of the lower first molars, and may require a fixed appliance as a result.

### *Forward Movement of Lower Second Molars*

The forward movement of lower second molars is not easily achieved. When the lower second molars have already tilted mesially and rolled lingually following the extraction of lower first molars, the aim of treatment is initially to upright the teeth and then to move them forward bodily.

A plane archwire of 0·40 mm diameter is used first to commence

124

correction of the mesiolingual inclination of the lower second molars. This archwire is expanded across the intermolar distance by at least 10 mm. Depending upon the inclination of the molars, anchorage or toe-in bends will probably not be required initially. The distal ends of the archwire are not turned down as they emerge from the molar tubes, so that the molars are free to tip distally.

Mesial movement of lower second molars is best achieved by using a combination of inter- and intramaxillary traction. The archwire is made of 0·40 or 0·45 mm diameter wire, and expanded across the intermolar width. The molars must move forward along the archwire under the influence of the traction which is applied.

Class II intermaxillary traction elastics are attached to mesiolingual hooks on the lower second molar bands, so helping to correct lingual or mesial inclination of these teeth.

Intramaxillary traction can be applied by elastics or coil springs. Elastics are attached mesially to archwire hooks lying in front of the lower canines, and distally to mesiobuccal hooks on the molar bands. Coil springs are compressed using a long ligature which is tied back to the mesiobuccal hooks on the molar bands.

Archwire closing loops placed immediately distal to the lower second premolar brackets can be used to apply intramaxillary traction. They have disadvantages, however; they increase the flexibility of the distal part of the archwire so that a certain amount of control over the molar is lost, and when activated they tend to rotate out of their intended position and cause irritation to neighbouring soft tissues.

When the degree of crowding in the lower arch is such that the space available following the extraction of first permanent molars is only just sufficient to allow alignment, the forward movement of the second permanent molars must be prevented, and Class II traction therefore not applied.

When the molars are forward into contact with the second premolars, a final archwire is required to produce uprighting. An

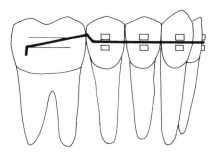

*Fig.* 12.6. Archwire, 0·45 mm, with vertical bayonet offset to over-correct 7| following forward movement into 6| space.

archwire with anchorage bends and vertical bayonet offsets is used (*Fig.* 12.6). Toe-in bends may also be necessary to correct rotation. The archwire can be activated progressively, but it is most important that the molar crown is prevented from moving distally. In order to prevent distal movement of the molar, the archwire can be turned down hard as it emerges from the molar tube, or a long ligature used to tie the molar forwards. Slight overtreatment with elevation of the mesial marginal ridge of the molar is desirable, and it is advisable to check the completion of movement with a radiograph because it is difficult to assess root paralleling clinically.

### Upper Molars

The forward movement of upper second molars is not as difficult to accomplish as forward movement of lower second molars. A satisfactory contact point between the second molar and second premolar may be established without the need for appliances.

The problem of providing sufficient anchorage commonly arises when the space provided by the extraction of upper first molars is required for the alignment of anterior teeth. If extra-oral traction is required it can be applied by means of an extra-oral arch fitting on the second molar bands. Sometimes it is difficult to make upper second molar bands retentive enough to withstand the forces generated by the extra-oral traction, which then has to be applied to the archwire or directly to the anterior teeth. If extra-oral traction is applied to the front of the archwire, stops must be placed in the archwire in front of the second molars to deliver the force of the extra-oral traction to the molars and to prevent them from moving forward along the archwire.

If the alignment of the premolars is satisfactory at the commencement of treatment, the best way of retracting them is to use a removable appliance, fitted over bands on the upper second molars. If, however, the premolars require rotation or buccolingual movement they must be banded and aligned before being moved distally into the first molar extraction space. Retraction of premolars in this instance is carried out with compressed coil springs, or elastic ligature, and this will of course consume some, or even all, of the first molar extraction space.

Rotation and tipping of upper second molars is not such a complication of forward movement as it is in the lower arch. Toe-in and uprighting bends may be used if necessary. Often these need not be incorporated until the final archwires are made.

## IMPACTED MOLARS

Occasionally a second molar impacts against a first molar and fails to erupt fully. Such teeth may be disimpacted using a small sectional

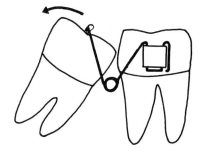

*Fig.* 12.7. Sectional arch to upright 7̅|.
The arch is attached to 6̅| by a pin and
tube system, and engages a pin inserted
into 7̅|.

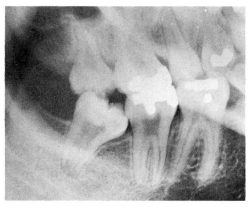

A

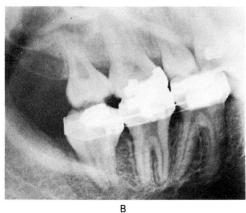

B

*Fig.* 12.8. Uprighted 8̅| with a sectional arch. A lower lingual arch to
bands on 6̅|6̅ was used to improve the anchorage. A, Before treatment.
B, 8̅7̅| have been banded and 8̅| apex brought forward.

127

arch from a band on the first molar (*Fig.* 12.7). A lingual arch is also necessary to increase the anchorage if other teeth further forward in the arch are not banded. The sectional arch is attached to the molar by means of a McKeag box and it is usually necessary to insert a pin into the occlusal surface of the second molar to engage the end of the sectional arch. When the impacted tooth has been moved distally it is generally possible to band the tooth and then to upright it conventionally (*Fig.* 12.8).

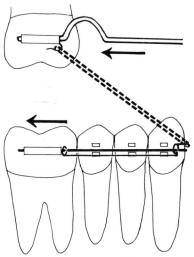

*Fig.* 12.9. Extra-oral force transmitted to $\overline{6|6}$ by means of Class III traction to a sliding jig.

## DISTAL MOVEMENT OF LOWER MOLARS

This movement is difficult to achieve without a complex appliance system. Slight distal movement may be obtained using a lower lingual arch which is activated to push the molar distally. The reaction to this movement tends to procline the lower incisors, and this is usually undesirable. Whilst extra-oral traction can be applied directly to the lower molars with an extra-oral arch, patients find it difficult to wear. It is therefore best applied to upper molar bands, and the extra-oral force transmitted indirectly to the lower arch with Class III intermaxillary traction. The elastics are attached to the anterior end of a 'sliding jig', which then presses against the molar tube (*Fig.* 12.9).

### REFERENCES

Reynolds L. M. (1976) *Br. J. Orthod.* **3**, 45.
Vig K. L. (1975) *Br. J. Orthod.* **2**, 217.

# CHAPTER 13

# ANCHORAGE

Anchorage is defined as 'the manner in which the reaction to applied forces is resisted' (British Standards Institute, 1969).

In clinical terms, 'anchorage' involves a consideration of the relationship between the applied force and available space. In some cases all the space gained by the extraction of teeth will be required for the alignment of the remaining teeth, in other cases only part of the extraction space will be required, whereas in a further group treatment is concerned with the closure of an excessive amount of space.

### Force and Tooth Movement

The magnitude of force required to move a tooth is related to:

1. Root area. The larger the root area the greater the force required. Thus first permanent molars require more applied force to produce movement than do lower incisors (*Fig.* 13.1).

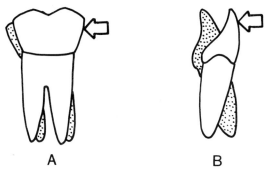

**A**          **B**

*Fig.* 13.1. A tipping force applied to a tooth with a large root area (A) produces less crown movement than when the same force is applied to a tooth with a small root area (B).

2. The quality of movement. If a tooth is free to tip in the direction of the applied force, then it will do so. The reason for this response is that the tooth moves in the direction of least resistance, a fulcrum of rotation being established (*Fig.* 13.2). If, however, the tooth is prevented from tipping and is compelled to move bodily, then more force is required to produce movement (the tooth is more resistant to

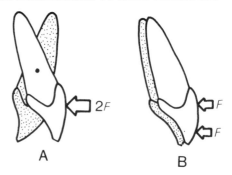

*Fig.* 13.2. When a tooth is free to tip in the direction of the applied force it will do so (A), and the amount of crown movement will exceed that which will occur when the same force is applied but the tooth prevented from tipping (B).

movement). Similarly, teeth subjected to torqueing or uprighting forces are more resistant to movement.

The rate of tooth movement is also related to the quality of movement taking place, and to root area. Teeth with relatively small root areas respond rapidly, and tipping movements are achieved more quickly than are bodily movements or torqueing.

### The Nature of Anchorage

When using orthodontic appliances Newton's third Law of Motion, 'Action and Reaction are equal and opposite' applies. This means that when a force is used to move a given group of teeth in one direction, an equal force will be applied in the opposite direction to the teeth providing the resistance against which the force is delivered (the anchor teeth). It is important to realize that this reciprocal force is likely to induce movement of the anchor teeth. To this extent, the concept of one group of teeth remaining static while another group moves is quite artificial. However, for descriptive purposes, teeth which comprise the site from which the force for intended tooth movement is delivered are referred to as anchor teeth (*Fig.* 13.3). The control of the movement of anchor teeth is of vital importance during the correction of malocclusion. To be more specific, it is important that there should be sufficient anchorage available. If, either because of faulty treatment planning or mechanics, there is insufficient anchorage, then the quality of result will be compromised. Appliance treatment is concerned with balancing opposed forces in such a manner that the desired tooth movements can be achieved.

The use of the words 'sufficient' and 'insufficient' in the context of

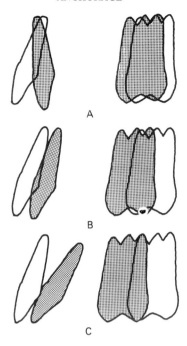

*Fig.* 13.3. Anchorage requirements for overjet reduction, indicated by the amount of forward movement of molars. A, Overjet reduction with simple tipping of incisors. B, Overjet reduction with bodily movement of incisors requires more anchorage. C, Overjet reduction with bodily movement of incisors and palatal torque of incisor apices requires even more anchorage.

anchorage implies that the amount of anchorage in a given circumstance can be assessed. This is indeed the case: groups of teeth possessing great resistance to movement are said to have a high anchorage value, and teeth which will move readily under the influence of an applied force are said to have a low anchorage value.

It has been explained previously that the force required to move a tooth is related to its root area, and to the quality of movement permitted. This fact, of course, applies equally to anchor teeth, and it is therefore possible to control within certain limits the amount of anchorage available in order to achieve the desired treatment result. The value of the anchorage in a given instance will depend upon:

1. The root area of the teeth comprising the anchorage unit.

2. The quality of permitted movement. Teeth which can only move bodily offer greater resistance than teeth which are free to tip.

When high forces are required for intended tooth movement over an extended period of time, maximum strain is placed upon the anchorage unit. Under these conditions the anchorage unit must be carefully planned so that it can provide the maximum resistance to movement.

Clinically, the value of the anchorage unit can be increased in the following ways when using fixed appliances:

1. Banding more teeth and incorporating them in the anchorage unit (so increasing the root area).

2. Using anchorage bends (so restricting tipping movements). Molar anchorage can be increased by the use of anchorage bends (*Fig.* 13.4). The bends are made in the archwire between the molar

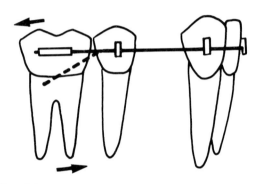

*Fig.* 13.4. Anchorage bends prevent mesial tipping of molars.

and premolar at approximately 30° to the occlusal plane. Anchorage bends prevent mesial tipping of the molars to which they are applied, and therefore make these teeth more resistant to forward movement. When placing an archwire incorporating anchorage bends it is important to ensure that the wire lies in the 12 o'clock position in the molar tube, otherwise rotation of the molar may be produced.

3. Use of uprighting and torqueing forces. If incisors are to be used as anchor teeth to resist a palatally or labially directed force, they offer more resistance if they must move bodily as a reaction to the applied force than if they are free to tip. The use of a torqueing archwire will make the incisors more resistant to a palatally directed force, and a reverse torqueing archwire will increase the anchorage value of the incisors against a buccally directed force. Similarly, uprighting forces can be used to make teeth more resistant to movement.

4. Palatal and lingual arches restrict tipping of molars and can therefore play a part in increasing anchorage value.

# REINFORCEMENT OF ANCHORAGE

## Intermaxillary Traction

Intermaxillary traction enables groups of teeth in one arch to provide anchorage for tooth movements in the opposing arch. With Class II traction, movement of teeth in the upper labial segment can be carried out using the lower buccal segments as anchorage. Depending upon the amount of extraction space available in the lower arch, the lower buccal segments can either be allowed to move forwards, or their movement restricted by using anchorage bends.

## Extra-oral Traction

Extra-oral traction is used to prevent forward movement of the upper buccal segments during alignment of the upper labial segments. In this manner molar teeth can be prevented from moving forward during distal movement of anterior teeth.

# ANCHORAGE PLANNING

Consider first the anchorage implications when an upper removable appliance is used to retract the upper canines (*Fig.* 13.5). A distally

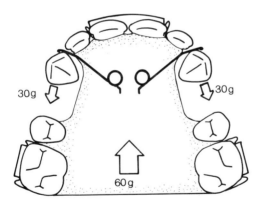

*Fig.* 13.5. When an upper removable appliance is used to retract 3|3 the force applied to retract these teeth is distributed to all the other teeth in contact with the base plate.

directed force of 30 g is applied to each canine, which will then tip distally. A mesially directed force of 60 g is therefore applied to the anchorage unit. The anchorage unit comprises 6521|1256 and the palatal mucosa in contact with the baseplate.

In such a case it might be expected that the upper canines will move

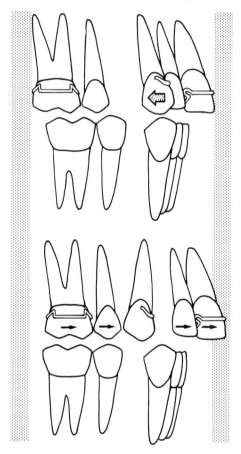

*Fig.* 13.6. Canine retraction with an upper removable appliance. 6521|
have moved forward as a reaction to distal movement of 3|.

distally with minimal forward movement of the anchorage unit, the
rationale being that whereas 30 g is sufficient to move a canine distally, 60 g is not sufficient to produce much forward movement of the
anchorage unit (the force applied to each anchor tooth being insufficient to produce significant movement).

What is the characteristic of the anchorage in this case which
makes it relatively resistant to movement? There are two factors:

1. The palatal acrylic bearing against the mucosa. (Fixed
appliances cannot depend upon anchorage from this source.)

2. The number of teeth in the anchorage unit. The important factor
here is the root area. The force per unit root area should be so low that

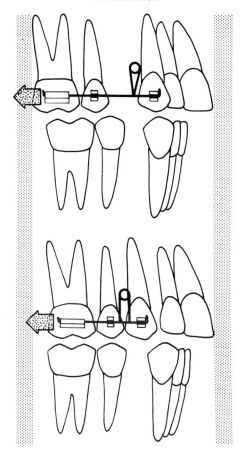

*Fig.* 13.7. Bodily canine retraction with a rectangular sectional archwire. 65| have moved forward as a reaction to distal movement of 3|. The arrows illustrate a distal force applied to 6|6 using E.O.T.

movement of the anchor teeth will be minimal.

In this example the anchorage value is high in comparison with the resistance of the canines to distal movement. Since the canines are free to tip distally they will offer relatively little resistance, and movement will occur relatively rapidly. Furthermore, a light force (30 g) is being used.

Even in the situation described, some forward movement of the anchorage unit must be expected. Such forward movement is described as anchorage loss, and is detectable as forward movement of 65|56 and an increase in overjet (*Fig.* 13.6.) It is important to recognize that if the canine retraction force is increased, then the force per unit root area on the anchor teeth is increased proportionally, and further anchorage loss will ensue. If there is excessive forward movement of the anchorage unit then the canines will not be retracted sufficiently to allow enough space for incisor realignment.

A fixed appliance mechanism designed to produce bodily retraction of upper canines is illustrated in *Fig.* 13.7. The upper first premolars have been extracted. This example should be compared with the case described above in which a removable appliance was used to move upper canines distally.

If upper canines are compelled to move bodily, then:

1. Greater force will need to be applied than if the teeth were free to tip distally.

2. The movement will be slower than if free tipping were allowed.

The anchorage requirement of such movement is thus considerable, and the risk of anchorage loss is great. The anchorage value of 65|56 is increased by preventing them from tipping mesially. This is achieved by using a relatively rigid archwire and brackets which do not allow the teeth to tip along the archwire. Even when the anchorage value has been increased in the manner described, mesial movement of the anchor unit must still be expected (*Fig.* 13.7). Excessive forward movement of the anchor teeth can be prevented by using extra-oral traction, which will apply a distal force to the upper molars.

It is important to recognize that it may not always be desirable to prevent forward movement of the anchor teeth. The amount of forward movement permissable will depend upon the distance the canines are to be retracted and the amount of space available. Anchorage reinforcement will be required when forward movement of the posterior teeth would prevent alignment of the anterior teeth. Anchor teeth must not be considered as immovable; in fact the possibility of controlled movement of anchor teeth is one of the principal advantages of using fixed appliances.

Consider now a Class II, division 1 case in which all four first premolars have been extracted, the aim of treatment being to reduce the overjet completely (*Fig.* 13.8). A fixed appliance is used, and intramaxillary traction applied to reduce the overjet, allowing the upper incisors and canines to tip distally.

The anchorage value of 65|56 must be sufficient to allow complete reduction of the overjet, not forgetting that some anchorage loss must be anticipated. If, taking into account the amount of space available, no anchorage loss can be permitted, then the anchorage must be reinforced; for example, by using extra-oral traction. An alternative approach would be to use intermaxillary traction, thereby employing the anchorage afforded by the lower molars and premolars to resist the distally directed tipping force applied to the upper labial segment

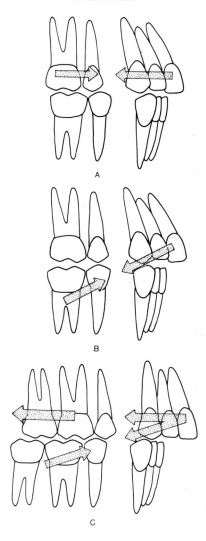

A

B

C

*Fig.* 13.8. A, A Class II, division 1 malocclusion in which the overjet can be reduced by tipping 21|12 using intramaxillary traction. B, A Class II, division 1 malocclusion in which the overjet can be reduced by tipping 21|12 using intermaxillary force. C, A severe Class II, division 1 malocclusion in which bodily retraction of 21|12 is required. Maximum anchorage is obtained by banding $\frac{7|7}{7|7}$ and extra-oral, intra-

maxillary, and intermaxillary traction should be used to reduce the overjet completely.

137

(*Fig.* 13.8B). Anchorage loss in this instance will be demonstrated by forward movement of the lower buccal segments with the potential risk of excessive forward movement in the lower arch. The possibility of using intermaxillary traction to provide anchorage in one arch for tooth movement in the other is a further advantage of using fixed appliances. The use of intermaxillary traction with removable appliances is severely restricted by problems of appliance retention.

If in the treatment of a Class II, division 1 malocclusion it is decided to reduce the overjet by bodily movement of the upper incisors in a palatal direction, the anchorage requirements are considerably increased (*Fig.* 13.8C). A further complication, which will make anchorage loss more likely, is the rate of movement of the incisors under these conditions. For a given amount of overjet reduction, treatment will be slower if bodily movement as opposed to tipping is required. In this instance the following methods of providing sufficient anchorage could be considered:

1. The use of extra-oral traction to prevent forward movement of the upper molars under the influence of intramaxillary traction. Alternatively, extra-oral traction could be applied directly to the archwire anteriorly.

2. Intermaxillary traction—providing space is available in the lower arch to accommodate the inevitable forward movement of the lower molars and premolars.

3. Use of anchorage bends to restrict forward movement of molars in both arches.

4. Banding of the upper second molars (and the lower second molars if intermaxillary traction is used) in order to increase the root area in the anchorage units.

It is sometimes necessary to close spaces by moving premolars and molars anteriorly. Under these conditions the teeth of the labial segment are considered as the anchor teeth. They may be made more resistant to movement and prevented from tipping in a palatal direction under the influence of the distally directed reciprocal force, by applying a torqueing archwire. In order to reduce anchorage requirements the molars and premolars are moved mesially one by one until all spaces are closed and axial inclinations corrected.

## Tooth Position and Anchorage

The factors which determine stability of tooth position are not fully understood. However, in describing the points which guide the operator in controlling tooth movement, we have adopted a dogmatic approach. This approach is based upon the concept of stability of the lower labial segment. We consider that this concept is best adopted whilst the operator gains experience with fixed appliances.

## The Lower Incisors

During treatment, the molar relationship, that is, the anteroposterior relationship of the upper and lower molars in occlusion, cannot be taken as a fixed reference point. Differential movement of molars during treatment is common, and frequently desirable.

The only *reference point* that can be used is the lower labial segment. The labiolingual position of the lower incisor crowns should for all practical purposes be the same at the end of treatment as it was at the start. This of course does not preclude alignment of lower incisors by correcting rotation and crowding, but no attempt is made to bring the angulation or labiolingual position of the lower incisors to a 'norm'. The reason for this is that the position of the crowns of the lower incisors is in large part determined by the lower lip and the tongue in a position of muscle balance. If the angulation of the lower incisors is altered by tipping, it is liable to relapse. The angulation of the upper incisors, on the other hand, can often be changed to reduce the overjet, by putting the crowns in a different soft-tissue environment (principally by altering their relationship with the lower lip).

It would be possible to gain space for the alignment of crowded lower incisors by proclining them on to a wider arc, or by maintaining their inclination but expanding the lower intercanine width. Unfortunately, both of these possibilities are liable to relapse, with recurrence of incisor crowding. Correct treatment of a crowded lower labial segment is distal movement of the lower canines away from the incisors, followed by alignment of the incisors without materially altering their labiolingual crown position.

If an alteration of the lower incisor axial inclination is suspected it is very useful to be able to assess this accurately with a lateral skull radiograph.

If the lower incisors have been proclined then there is not as much space available as there appears to be, for when the appliance is removed, the lower incisors are liable to retrocline to their original position.

## The Lower Canines

The position adopted by the lower canines when they have been moved far enough distally to provide enough room for incisor alignment becomes the point around which the upper labial and both buccal segments are arranged.

To enable complete reduction of overjet in a Class II, division 1 case the upper canines must in general be retracted into a Class I relationship to the expected final position of the lower canines. This may depend upon the upper buccal segments not having moved too far forward. Undue forward movement of the upper buccal segments is prevented by making them more resistant to movement.

139

Occasionally cases are encountered where there is a considerable disproportion between the sizes of upper and lower incisors. The aim of Class I canine relationship is not relevant in these cases, or in cases with retroclined upper incisors (Class II, division 2), where it is usually advisable to leave the upper canines in a half-unit Class II relationship rather than to retract them fully, if the angulation of the upper incisors is to be accepted.

### Class II Traction

The extent to which Class II traction can be used depends upon the amount of space remaining in the lower buccal segments when tooth alignment has been achieved. If there is no space available then Class II traction should not be used, or the whole lower arch may be moved forward and the lower incisors placed in an unstable position.

Consider the effect of Class II traction on a lower arch where forward movement of the lower buccal segments is required to close extraction spaces. It is presumed that lower first premolars have been extracted. The lower buccal segments will tend to move forward under the pull of the Class II traction. Because these teeth will not slide forward easily along the archwire some of the intermaxillary force is delivered through the archwire to the lower incisors, which are therefore in danger of being proclined. Intramaxillary traction in the lower arch, on the other hand, tends to retrocline the lower incisors, at the same time as bringing the lower buccal segments forwards. When Class II traction is used, intramaxillary traction may be necessary in the lower arch to prevent lower incisor proclination.

### Buccal Segment Relationship

If the extractions are symmetrical in opposing arches—for example, all first premolars—then at the end of treatment with all spaces closed the buccal segment relationship should be Class I with full cuspal interdigitation.

If the extractions in the opposing arches are not matched—for example, if upper first molars and lower first premolars are extracted—a Class I relationship of all the teeth in the buccal segments cannot be produced. This does not matter provided there is good cuspal interdigitation.

### Centre Lines

Commonly, the whole problem of anchorage control is complicated by a shift of centre line. If the lower centre line is to the left, for example, the right buccal segment and right canine usually follow to a certain extent. As a result, the right canine is foward, without necessarily being proclined forward of the lower incisors in the way classically associated with lower labial segment crowding. The unwary can retract both the lower canines sufficiently to relieve crowding, then correct the upper right canine into Class I with the lower right canine. This is a false position, as in fact the lower right canine should be retracted further in order to allow for correction of the lower centre line. Ideally, at the end of treatment the centre lines should be coincident, otherwise a satisfactory buccal segment interdigitation may be impossible to achieve.

## ANCHORAGE CONTROL

The control of tooth movement with fixed appliances is complicated, and involves balancing the movement of groups of teeth so that at the completion of treatment a satisfactory occlusal relationship is produced.

The amount of anchorage necessary to enable the required tooth movement to be produced can only be assessed if the precise aims of treatment with regard to tooth position are defined before treatment is started. A clear picture of the expected final occlusal result is of great importance. When the extraction of teeth is being considered at the treatment-planning stage, the amount of space which a given combination of extractions will provide should be considered in relation to the anchorage which will be required to produce the desired tooth movement.

When the treatment plan has been decided, the mechanical problems of producing the desired occlusal result can be considered. They are concerned with balancing the anchorage values of groups of teeth—in other words, making groups of teeth more or less resistant to movement. The difficulties of anchorage control continue throughout treatment and can only be overcome if the operator:

1. Has a clear picture of the desired final occlusion.
2. Is fully aware of tooth movements occurring between visits.
3. Understands the mechanical principles involved in the functioning of the appliance.

## REFERENCES

Fletcher G. G. T. (1961) *Trans. Br. Soc. Study Orthod. 31.*
Haack D. C. (1963) *Am. J. Orthod.* **49,** 330.
Mills J. R. E. (1967) *Trans. Br. Soc. Study Orthod.* **54,** 11.
Mills J. R. E. (1970) *The Orthodontist* **2,** 32.
Sandusky W. C. (1965) *Am. J. Orthod.* **51,** 262.
Sims M. R. (1971) *Am. J. Orthod.* **59,** 456.
Storey E. and Smith R. (1952) *Aust. J. Dent.* **56,** 11.

# CHAPTER 14

# FINISHING PROCEDURES

## RETENTION

Experience has shown that in most cases, if appliances are removed as soon as tooth movement is completed, a variable amount of relapse in tooth position will occur.

The causes of such relapse are often difficult to identify because the factors which determine stability are not easily quantified. The form and behaviour of the surrounding soft tissues are certainly an important factor. If the teeth have been moved into positions in which they are subjected to muscular forces which are not 'in balance' the teeth will move under the influence of the applied forces. It is thus pointless to move teeth into a position of muscular imbalance and then retain them in that position, hoping that no relapse will occur when the appliance is finally removed. Likewise it can be argued that if teeth have been moved into a position of 'balance' with regard to the soft-tissue forces, no retention whatsoever is required.

While an appreciation of the role of soft-tissue factors in determining tooth position is important, the precise effects of muscular forces upon teeth at the completion of treatment are very difficult to predict. A further complication is that soft-tissue factors are by no means the only factors which determine tooth position. The fibres of the periodontal membrane, alveolar bone, and gingivae may also be instrumental in causing relapse. Certain of these fibres have been associated with rotational relapse, and others may be connected with relapse of apical position. During the period of retention these fibres are able to reorganize their position relative to the teeth, and the possibility of relapse is then reduced.

Occlusal factors, which again are difficult to measure, are also important in determining tooth position. If, when the teeth are in occlusion, opposing cuspal inclines relate in such a way that displacing forces are generated, an alteration of tooth position may occur. Ideally, at the completion of tooth movement, the manner in which the upper teeth relate to the lower teeth in occlusion should not cause displacing forces to be delivered to teeth in either arch.

### The Principle of Overcorrection

Certain tooth movements have been found to be liable to relapse despite prolonged retention. Rotational movement and apical movement are notable in this connexion. It has been found that if these movements are 'overcorrected' and the teeth then retained in that position, relapse to the initial tooth position is less likely to occur.

## Rotational Overcorrection

One method which has been used for the alignment of a rotationally displaced tooth is not merely to rotate it into alignment, but to 'overrotate' it and then to retain it in that position for an extended period (perhaps one year). The amount of overrotation required to prevent relapse towards the original rotational displacement may be as much as 100 per cent—in other words, if a tooth is rotated 20° clockwise it should be overrotated to 20° anticlockwise. It is then anticipated that the inevitable relapse following appliance removal will result in the tooth assuming a satisfactory rotational position, in line with neighbouring teeth.

The treatment of severe rotations in this way is time consuming and may prevent or delay the alignment of other teeth.

## Pericision

Although this technique has only relatively recently been described and long-term results are not available, the authors consider that its importance is such that it merits a short description in this book. The evidence suggests that pericision reduces the likelihood of rotational relapse. In addition, it would seem that overrotation, at least to 100 per cent, is not so important, and the period of retention can be considerably reduced.

Work by Reitan (1959) suggests that the free gingival and transseptal fibres of the periodontal membrane are causative agents in the relapse of rotated teeth. The relatively minor surgical procedure known as pericision is concerned with sectioning these fibres.

Under local anaesthetic, a number 11 scalpel blade is used to separate the free gingival and trans-septal fibres from the rotated tooth. The blade is inserted through the gingival crevice in an apical direction, to the crest of the alveolar bone. Care should be taken to ensure that the blade is taken completely round the neck of the tooth to the depth of the alveolar bone crest. To date, there is no evidence to suggest that there is any permanent damage to the periodontal tissues following this procedure.

It is recommended that teeth which have been 'pericised' in this way should be retained in their position for six months, following which the appliance can be removed.

## Archwires for Retention

The function of the archwire during the period of retention is to hold the teeth rigidly in the positions into which they have been moved.

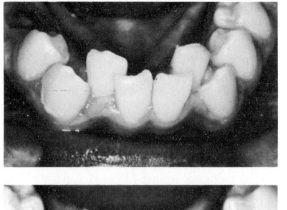

A

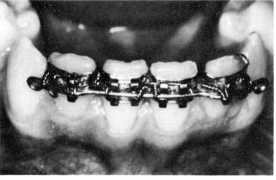

B

*Fig.* 14.1. A, Crowded lower incisors before treatment. B, A sectional retainer to maintain position of 2|2.

Retaining archwires are therefore made in 0·45, 0·50, or 0·55 mm diameter wire. Because of the relative inflexibility of these archwires they must be very carefully prepared in order to prevent inadvertent tooth movement during the period of retention. Full bracket engagement must be possible without distorting the archwire from its passive form. The teeth are then ligated tightly to the archwire.

Archwire offsets are used to retain overcorrection of rotational and apical position (*Fig.* 14.1). When a space between two teeth has been closed, reopening of the space during the period of retention can be prevented by archwire stops, or by tying the teeth together with a long ligature. If an overjet has been reduced, proclination of the upper incisors can be prevented by turning the end of the upper archwire upwards hard against the distal end of the molar tube, or by tying the archwire back to the molars with long ligatures.

Edgewise sectional retaining archwires can be used to maintain the overcorrected rotational and apical position of teeth which have been aligned using edgewise brackets. Edgewise sectional archwires are sometimes used in this way to retain the position of lower incisors and canines. The relative rigidity of the rectangular archwire and the possibility of control of tooth position which it affords make it particularly suitable for the construction of sectional retaining archwires.

Certain tooth movements, for instance diastema closure and the correction of severe rotations, require prolonged or even permanent retention. Such retention can be provided by spurs or staples made from 0·30 mm wire bonded into small cavities in the palatal aspect of the teeth concerned (*Fig.* 14.2). The wire is bonded in position using

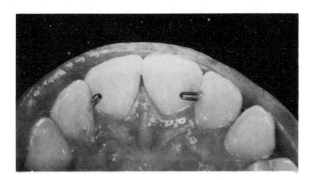

*Fig.* 14.2. Stainless-steel spurs bonded into 2|2 for prolonged retention of rotations.

an acid-etch technique and provides positive and aesthetically satisfactory retention.

### Band Removal

When removing bands, great care must be taken not to cause damage to the teeth. The enamel of the incisal edges of incisor teeth is particularly liable to fracture during band removal. The correct pliers, suitably protected with cotton-wool rolls or soft synthetic facings, should be used, and excessive forces never applied. Incisor band-removing pliers carrying cutting edges which split the band facilitate band removal and make damage to teeth less likely. Lower incisor bands may be particularly difficult to remove. It is sometimes necessary to split these bands with a bur, taking care, of course, not to damage the tooth surface.

After band removal the teeth should be scaled and polished to remove any remnants of cement adhering to the tooth surface. A thorough examination for carious cavities should then be made, and arrangements made for any necessary conservation treatment.

## Removable Appliances for Retention

Removable appliances can be used to retain tooth position following fixed-appliance treatment. However, it is not possible to retain apical or rotational position rigidly with removable appliances. An upper removable appliance with cribs on upper first molars, and a reverse-loop labial bow running from the distal of |3 to the distal of 3|, can be used to retain overjet reduction and prevent reopening of spaces between teeth. The labial bow can be adjusted to retain rotational overcorrection, but the teeth are not held as rigidly as when a fixed appliance is used. The thickness of the band material is such that when the bands are removed spaces are left between the teeth. These spaces can be closed by activation of a removable retainer. Removable retaining appliances have the advantage that they can be slowly discarded over a period of time, so allowing the occlusion to 'settle' to a certain extent during the period of part-time retention.

### Tooth Positioners

Tooth positioners are flexible one-piece plastic appliances which fit over the crowns of the teeth in both upper and lower arches. They are used as retaining appliances, and they may also be constructed in such a way as to produce a limited amount of tooth movement.

Tooth positioners are prepared on models made from impressions taken at the end of active treatment. Where necessary, teeth are sectioned from the models and their position altered slightly before the positioner is made. Positioners prevent the patient from eating and talking and they are therefore usually worn only at night.

### REFERENCES

Edwards J. G. (1970) *Am. J. Orthod.* **57,** 35.
Reitan K. (1959) *Angle Orthod.* **29,** 105.
Riedel R. A. (1969) In: Graber T. M. (ed.) *Current Orthodontic Concepts and Techniques,* vol. 2. Philadelphia, Saunders.
Strahan J. D. and Mills J. R. E. (1969) *Trans. Br. Soc. Study Orthod.* **56,** 91.
Wells N. E. (1970) *Am. J. Orthod.* **58,** 351.

CHAPTER 15

# THE DEVELOPMENT OF FIXED APPLIANCES

Orthodontic tooth movement has been carried out for many hundreds of years, the first descriptions of tooth movement dating to a few years B.C.

Modern fixed-appliance treatment can be traced back to a Frenchman, P. Fauchard, who made a buccally placed metal arch to which teeth were individually ligated by means of fibrous ligatures. This 'bandalette' appliance was described in 1726, and it enabled crude alignment of the teeth to be achieved by means of expansion of the dental arch.

Schangé invented a band in 1841 that was fitted to the teeth by means of a clamp which was adjustable to accommodate different sized teeth. Bands were also made from precious metals, copper, and brass. In 1871 Magill first used dental cement to attach a band to a tooth. Extra-oral forces were first described by Kingsley in 1866, and intermaxillary traction (Baker Anchorage) was used late in the nineteenth century. By that time the need for greater control over tooth movement led to the development of attachments which were soldered to the lingual aspect of the bands, enabling misplaced teeth to be ligated to a buccal archwire. These attachments were single spurs which prevented the ligature wires slipping, and allowed some rotational control. Brass ligatures were used, and progressively tightened as the teeth moved.

At that stage of development there was no attempt to correct malocclusions by placing teeth in a stable soft-tissue environment. Angle's conviction was that if teeth were moved into their correct occlusal relationship stability would be assured. Angle's early appliances had buccal tubes soldered to molar bands, and a buccal expansion arch which was activated by screws. Malpositioned teeth were banded and tied onto the arch. Tooth movements took place by tipping.

## The Development of Controlled Root Movement

Angle was well aware of the value of bodily movement of molars to aid anchorage, and in 1912 he described the pin and tube appliance, which was the first appliance capable of root movement, as opposed to simple tipping (*Fig.* 15.1A). The pin and tube appliance described by Angle was very difficult to use, because a high degree of precision was required to fabricate the archwire. Despite its limitations,

147

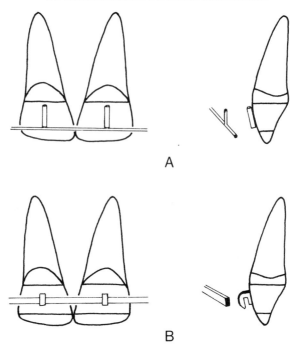

*Fig.* 15.1. A, Pin and tube appliance. B, Ribbon arch appliance.

however, the pin and tube appliance was an outstanding advance in that it showed the way towards greater control over tooth movement.

The ribbon arch appliance was described by Angle in 1916 (*Fig.* 15.1B). A precision bracket was attached to the bands with a channel that accepted a rectangular archwire. This was the first use of rectangular section wires, and adjustments could be made so as to produce accurate repositioning of roots. About 10 years later Angle described the edgewise mechanism in which pinched and soldered bands were fitted to most of the teeth. The rectangular archwire was now inserted into the brackets with the longer dimension horizontal —hence the term edgewise. The archwire was held into the bracket by ligatures, and eyelets were soldered onto the bands to aid in the correction of rotations. Treatment was still based on a non-extraction philosophy of arch expansion.

*Johnson Twin-wire Appliance*

The forces generated by the early edgewise mechanisms were very high, and in the 1930s Johnson introduced the twin-wire arch, which was designed to produce lighter tooth-moving forces. Two light buccal round archwires were used in combination to achieve rotation and alignment of the upper incisors. In the original technique special brackets were devised, and Class II traction was used to a lower lingual arch. An advantage of the Johnson twin-wire arch was its ability to correct incisor displacement with the minimum of bands.

The twin-wire arch is constructed of two 0·25 mm diameter hard stainless-steel wires drawn into end tubes of 0·90 mm outside diameter. The arch is thus rigid in the buccal segments and flexible in the labial segment.

Where there are considerable rotational or labiolingual displacements, partial engagements of the arch is indicated at the commencement of alignment. It is also possible to engage only one of the twin wires in the bracket in order to reduce the force applied (*Fig. 15.2*). The twin-wire arch can be used with edgewise brackets.

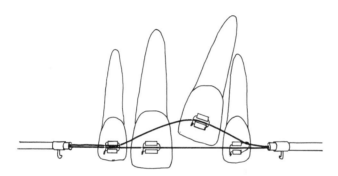

*Fig.* 15.2. Twin-wire arch showing engagement of only one wire in ⌊1 bracket.

Overrotation of teeth requires the use of spurs or wings on the bands. Alternatively a small piece of stainless-steel tubing may be held under the archwire next to the bracket by means of the ligature which holds the archwire in the bracket.

The twin-wire section of the arch suffers permanent distortion fairly readily and an arch will often need replacement before satisfactory alignment is achieved.

The twin-wire arch can also be used for overjet reduction using intermaxillary or intramaxillary elastics hooked onto the hooks at the medial aspect of the end tubes.

Developments of the edgewise technique have continued, with many variations on bracket design, and the use of more flexible archwires. Tweed was the first person to use the edgewise technique in conjunction with extractions, and his treatment method forms the basis of many of today's edgewise techniques.

## Labiolingual Appliances

At about the same time as Angle was beginning to use the edgewise mechanism, Mershon developed the lingual arch. Relatively rigid mandibular, and maxillary lingual arches were attached to molar bands. These arches carried springs that produced tooth movement by tipping. Their action was similar to that of the modern removable appliance. The lower arch was used for tooth movements in the upper arch, by means of Class II elastic traction. There was little concern, however, for the proclination of the lower incisors which frequently occurred.

The use of labial and lingual arches became popular because of the relative ease with which they could be fabricated and adjusted. From a mechanical point of view the labiolingual technique, as it was called, offered much less control over tooth position than the edgewise technique. At the present time the labiolingual appliance has been largely superseded by the modern removable appliance as a result of the use of new materials (acrylic and stainless-steel), and the development of the Adams clasp.

## Light-wire Techniques

The use of light forces in fixed appliance techniques, of which the Johnson twin-wire appliance is an early example, has continued to the present day. The Begg appliance which was originally described in 1956 is an example of a light wire technique, which uses round archwires exclusively. The Begg bracket resembles Angle's original ribbon arch bracket. The Begg system is an extraction-based philosophy, and uses intra-oral anchorage exclusively.

The trend in edgewise techniques is to use lighter round archwires for initial tooth movements, keeping the thicker rectangular archwires for the later stages of treatment.

# CHAPTER 16

# ADVANCED TECHNIQUES

A number of specific fixed-appliance techniques have been developed. Each of these 'advanced techniques' demands the use of a particular design of bracket and archwire. Furthermore, each technique specifies treatment objectives and diagnostic criteria, so that a total 'philosophy' of treatment is implied.

These techniques require a high degree of skill in wire bending and meticulous attention to detail during treatment. For this reason they should only be used if the operator has undergone a practical course of instruction in the particular treatment method.

Because of the precise manner in which the magnitude and direction of force can be applied, there is evidence to suggest that stable changes in dental base relationship and soft-tissue profile can be achieved by experienced operators using these techniques. Bodily movement of both upper and lower incisors is possible, and stable alterations in the position of the lower labial segment can be produced. However, for the postgraduate student of orthodontics, we believe that the concept of stability of the lower labial segment (*see* Chapter 13) is valuable, and that cases appearing to require alteration of lower labial segment position should be undertaken only by the experienced operator.

A brief description of the main techniques, covering their principal features, is included here so that the reader can be aware of complex techniques in use at the present time.

## *Edgewise Techniques*

There are a number of techniques based upon the use of edgewise brackets and deriving from the original work of Dr. Angle. Rectangular section archwires are not necessarily used throughout treatment. In some techniques they are used only in the final stages of treatment, earlier tooth movement having been carried out using round archwires, which provide greater flexibility.

Several variations of the standard single edgewise bracket are used. Two archwire channel sizes are in common use—0·022 in (0·55 mm) and 0·018 in (0·45 mm). These dimensions refer to the occlusogingival measurement. The size of channel used is a matter of personal choice, some operators preferring the 0·022 in (0·55 mm) channel because it will accommodate the more rigid rectangular archwires over 0·018 in (0·45 mm). Siamese brackets enable a more efficient force couple to be applied for rotating and uprighting, but the span of archwire between adjacent teeth is reduced with consequent reduction in flexibility. Brackets in which the archwire channel is angled are used by some orthodontists to apply torqueing forces without having to place torqueing bends in the archwire.

The Tweed technique, developed by Charles H. Tweed, is the classic edgewise technique of North America. Single 0·022 in (0·55 mm) slot edgewise brackets are used, with mesial and distal eyelets to facilitate rotation, and the molar bands are fitted with matching rectangular buccal tubes. Second permanent molars may be banded early in treatment in order to maximize available anchorage. Round archwires are used initially in order to facilitate bracket levelling and the correction of gross displacements, but the more rigid rectangular archwires are commonly used to produce canine retraction.

The concept of 'Ideal Arch Form' is used as a basis for archwire design. Accurate measurements of arch length and tooth width are taken. These measurements are used to construct the Bonwill Hawley Arch Graph which is then used as a template for successive archwire fabrication. Three 'orders' of bend are identified (*Fig.* 16.1). The

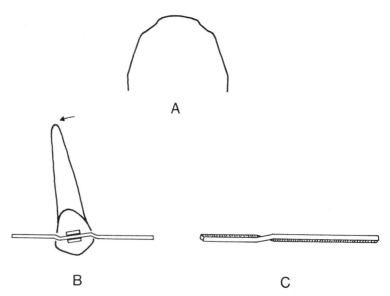

*Fig.* 16.1. A, First-order bends are made in the horizontal plane. B, Second-order bends are made in a vertical plane, at right angles to the occlusal plane. C, Third-order bends: this term is used in conjunction with rectangular wire only and refers to bends made longitudinally along the wire, thus twisting the wire.

technique is capable of producing excellent results with very precise tooth repositioning. Intra-oral anchorage is supplemented by the use of extra-oral traction in order to achieve the treatment aims prescribed at the diagnostic stage.

The rationale of diagnosis and treatment planning is peculiar to the Tweed technique. Serial lateral skull radiographs are used in a cephalometric analysis to identify growth trends. Growth trend classification and the Diagnostic Facial Triangle are used to indicate precise treatment aims and the timing of treatment. Permanent teeth are extracted if necessary in order that treatment aims can be achieved. Great attention is paid to facial aesthetics. Harmonious facial aesthetics are considered as being dependent upon a 'normal' relationship of the dental arches to the jaw bones and head structures.

## Begg Technique

The Begg Technique, developed by Dr P. R. Begg and first described in the 1950's is now widely used. Like the Tweed technique it is capable of producing excellent results, but the two techniques are fundamentally different in respect of diagnostic criteria and mechanism. The round archwire is located loosely in the Begg bracket, so that teeth are free to tip under the influence of applied forces. The freedom of teeth to move in a controlled manner with relation to the archwire is a basic feature of the mechanism. Apical movements are achieved by using accessory springs.

The use of Begg technique depends upon the banding of teeth in both arches so that intermaxillary traction elastics can be used. The extraction of four permanent teeth is usually required, and, in its pure form, Begg technique does not require the use of extra-oral traction. The Begg appliance utilizes the 'differential light force concept' whereby groups of teeth are made more or less resistant to movement according to the magnitude, duration, and direction of applied forces. 'Light' (flexible) round archwires are used, particularly in the early stages of treatment, and vertical loops are incorporated in order that full engagement of the archwire in the brackets can be obtained without applying excessive forces.

The two techniques described above illustrate fundamentally different mechanical approaches. The Tweed technique uses edgewise brackets, and the greater part of treatment is achieved using rectangular archwires. Tipping of teeth along and around the rectangular archwire is largely prevented because of the bracket and archwire combination. On the other hand, the Begg technique employs a bracket and archwire combination which allows teeth to tip with relation to the round archwire. The edgewise mechanism enables teeth to be tipped, torqued, and rotated by suitable activation of the rectangular archwire; whereas in the Begg technique accessory springs are required to produce torqueing and uprighting. The Tweed technique depends upon the use of extra-oral traction, whereas the Begg technique uses intra-oral anchorage only.

Other techniques have been developed which combine certain aspects of the edgewise and Begg methods. Attempts have been made to unite in a single technique the simplicity and precision of the edgewise bracket–rectangular archwire combination, and the rapid unravelling which is seen when using light forces of the Begg mechanism. In the light-wire appliance described by Jarabak the bracket used is basically of the edgewise type, incorporating a rectangular archwire channel. However, a large part of treatment is achieved using relatively small diameter light wires incorporating carefully positioned vertical and horizontal helices and loops. The anterior teeth carry modified brackets with vertical slots, enabling round archwires to produce tipping, rotation, and bodily movements.

In the 'Combination Technique' of Fogel and McGill a Siamese edgewise bracket incorporating a vertical slot is used. The technique was developed using a bracket which is intended to confer the benefits of the Begg single point contact bracket with the possibility of changing to a rectangular archwire in the later stages of treatment. During the first stage of treatment a 'bracket insert' is placed in the vertical bracket channel. This insert incorporates a narrow slot into which small-diameter round multilooped archwires can be placed to produce gentle movement by tipping. In the second stage the insert is discarded, and round archwires used in the edgewise channel. Finally, rectangular archwires are placed in the 'edgewise stage'.

The 'progressive light edgewise technique' described by Ricketts does not demand the banding of all teeth in both arches at the beginning of treatment. Banding is carried out progressively throughout treatment, and removable appliances may be used in the early stages. Archwire flexibility is obtained by the incorporation of loops and helices, and archwire fabrication is simplified by using preformed items. The bracket is a modification of the edgewise bracket with angled archwire channel so that torque forces are applied when using rectangular archwires, without the need to place torqueing bends.

## Future Developments

There is no technique that is without its disadvantages. There are currently many differing kinds of bracket and treatment method. Future developments in materials will no doubt simplify fixed-appliance technique and bring about greater mechanical efficiency, but careful attention to detail and precise monitoring of the tooth movements that are taking place will always be essential to achieve a first-class result.

## REFERENCES

Begg P. R. and Kesling P. C. (1977) *Begg Orthodontic Theory and Technique,* 3rd ed. Philadelphia, Saunders.

Fogel M. S. and Magill J. M. (1972) *The Combination Technique in Orthodontic Practice.* Philadelphia, Lippincott.

Jarabak J. R. and Fizzell B. S. (1972) *Technique and Treatment with Light-wire Appliances.* St Louis, Mosby.

Senior W. B. (1975) *Br. J. Orthod.* **2,** 7, 105, 149.

Tweed C. H. (1966) *Clinical Orthodontics* (2 vols). St Louis, Mosby.

# GENERAL BIBLIOGRAPHY

**STANDARD TEXTBOOKS**

Adams C. P. (1977) *The Design and Construction of Removable Orthodontic Appliances,* 4th ed. Bristol, Wright.

Begg P. R. and Kesling P. C. (1977) *Orthodontic Theory and Technique,* 2nd ed. Philadelphia, Saunders.

Graber T. M. (ed.) (1975) *Current Orthodontic Concepts and Techniques.* 2nd ed. Philadelphia, Saunders.

Houston W. J. B. (1976) *Orthodontic Diagnosis.* Bristol, Wright.

Houston W. J. B. and Isaacson K. G. (1977) *Orthodontic Treatment with Removable Appliances.* Bristol, Wright.

Tweed C. H. (1976) *Clinical Orthodontics* (2 vols). St. Louis, Mosby.

# APPENDIX 1

The following list, which is *not* comprehensive, gives the names and addresses of some of the suppliers of orthodontic equipment which may be used when working with fixed appliances.

## DENTAURUM

7530 Pforzheim,
Postfach 440,
West Germany.

Hawley, Russell & Baker,
35 Darkes, Lane,
Potters Bar,
Hertfordshire.
Tel. 0707–55579.

## ORMCO

Ormco Corporation,
1332 South Lone Hill Avenue,
Glendora,
California 91740, U.S.A.

Oradent Ltd,
88A High Street,
Eton
Windsor
Berkshire SL4 6AF
Tel. 07535–57714

## ROCKY MOUNTAIN

Rocky Mountain Dental Products Co.,
P.O. Box 1887,
Denver,
Colorado 80201, U.S.A.

Orthodontic Products
Sheffield Ltd,
550 Oxford St.
Sheffield S6 3FG
Tel. 0742–662654

## T.P.

T. P. Laboratories Inc.,
P.O. Box 73,
La Porte,
Indiana 46350, U.S.A.

TRI Services,
P.O. Box 52,
Driebergen,
Holland.

## UNITEK

Unitek Corporation
950 Royal Oakes Drive,
Monrovia,
California, U.S.A.

Orthomax Dental Ltd,
Carr House,
Carrbottom Road,
Bradford BD5 9BJ,
Tel. 0274–33842.

## IN THE UNITED KINGDOM

*ORTHODONTIC PLIERS* are also available from:

Claudius Ash Sons & Co. Ltd,
Amalco House,
26–40 Broadwick Street,
London W1A 2AD.
Tel. 01–437 4333.

*STAINLESS-STEEL WIRE AND TAPES* can be obtained from:

K. C. Smith,
Redbrook Road,
Monmouth
Gwent.

# INDEX